YOU AND YOUR DI

By the same author :

- जीवन मधुमेह के संग
- हृदय रोग और आपः रोग, उपचार एवं सावधानियाँ
- Diet And Diabetes
- You And Your Diabetes

About the Author

Dr. A.K. Jhingan, (*b.* 1949) M.B.B.S., M.D. Medicine, is working as Senior Consultant, Physician and Diabetologist in Jaipur golden Hospital and a visiting Physician in Sir Ganga Ram Hospital, Delhi. He is attached with State Bank of India as a Senior Physician and Medical Advisor.

Author started working in field of Diabetes since 1983 and has been organizing diabetes Detection and Educational Camps in and around Delhi.

Author is a firm believer of the fact that Diabetics who know more about disease can live longer.

Author has written three books, 'You and Your Heart', Jeevan Madhumeh Ke Sang' and 'Hriday Rog aur Aap' (the last two books are in Hindi). These books have been appreciated by masses and this is evident from the fact that their new editions had to be brought out.

Delhi Diabetes Research Centre (DDRC) is a registered Society and was established by a group of eminent doctors from India and abroad. Diabetes educators and social workers. Its sole aim is to help and educated Diabetics by arranging regular seminars and conferences, so that they can lead normal life. So far DDRC has organized more than 105 such camps in and around Delhi.

3rd Revised & Enlarged Edition

You
and
Your Diabetes

Dr. A.K. Jhingan

M.B.B.S., M.D. (Medicine), FIAMS

Director

Delhi Diabetes Research Centre (DDRC)

&

President

Juvenile Diabetes Association of India

CONCEPT PUBLISHING COMPANY, NEW DELHI-110059

Cataloging in Publication Data—DK
Courtesy: D.K. Agencies (P) Ltd. <docinfo@dkagencies.com>

Jhingana, E. Ke. (Aśoka Ke.), 1949-
    You and your diabetes / A.K. Jhingan.
    — 3rd rev. & enl. ed.
    p. cm.
    ISBN 8180691519

    1. Diabetes.   I. Title.

DDC 616.462   21

ISBN 81-8069-151-9

First Published 1998
Reprinted 2000
Revised and Enlarged Edition 2001
Third Revised and Enlarged Edition 2005

© Dr. A.K. Jhingan (b. 1949)

Published and Printed by
Ashok Kumar Mittal
Concept Publishing Company
A/15-16, Commercial Block, Mohan Garden
NEW DELHI - 110059 (India)

Phones : 25351460, 25351794
Fax : 091-11-25357103
Email : publishing@conceptpub.com

This book is
Dedicated
To
All the Scientists, Doctors, Nurses,
Social Workers and Individuals
who are Engaged in the
Welfare of Diabetic Patients

Do You Know?

- Diabetes is the fifth largest killer disease
- People with Diabetes have more problems like
  — Heart Troubles,
  — Paralytic Strokes,
  — Blindness,
  — Kidney Failure,
  — Sexual Problems, and
  — Frequent Infections.
- Majority of Diabetics think it is not a Major health problem.
- 80% Diabetic Patients are Unaware of the Complications of Diabetes.

Foreword

A person with Diabetes requires full information regarding various do's and donot's in everyday living.

It is very essential that Diabetics realize their own responsibilities in control of Blood Glucose and requirement of medications.

A person with Diabetes has to be aware of certain emergencies and in such events how these may be circumvented.

Dr. A.K. Jhingan has fulfilled the needful requirement of Diabetes in our country. In a very simple language and practical manner, view points of a Diabetologist are presented.

I sincerely hope that full use of this information is made by Diabetics.

M.M.S. Ahuja
Formerly Prof. and Head
Department of Endocrinology and
Metabolic Unit,
A.I.I.M.S.

Preface to the Second Edition

You and your Diabetes was published in 1998. The message of the new edition of this book is that Medical science moves forward and most of the questions stay the same but many of the answers have changed. The outlook for people with diabetes improves year by year.

One thing remains unchanged, the absolute necessity for people with diabetes to learn and understand as much as they can about their disease. Ignorance is often damaging and can sometimes be lethal. More information is available about prevention of prime factors which produce complications of Diabetes and new treatment modalities like, islet cell transplantation, pancrease cell transplantation, new ways of Insulin delivery system, i.e., pens and pumps and new group of oral medicines which reduce Insulin resistance and help in controlling blood sugar levels.

People with diabetes will also want to keep themselves up-to-date and well-informed and we hope this new edition will be of help to them.

Dr. Kamalesh Jhingan

Introduction

So many books about diabetes have been written and the reader gets more confused going through lengthy chapters about the disease. After discussing with many patients of Diabetes it was felt that there should be a book in simple language which should be interesting and informative.

Diabetes is a disease which can be very well controlled and one can lead a normal life. Complications of Diabetes can make the life of Diabetic miserable due to Blindness, Kidney failure, Neuritis and Paralysis.

Recently a study was conducted in insulin dependent Diabetic patients and according to it, if these patients keep their blood sugar under control then blindness can be prevented in the 76% of such patients, kidney failure in 35 to 56% of such Diabetic patients and Neuritis Nerve involvement in 60% of such Diabetic patients.

Intensive control of Diabetes Mellitus decreases the rate of complications, improves the patients quality of life, and decreases the total cost of care associated with both type I and type II Diabetes. Study, the United Kingdom Prospective Diabetes Study (UKPDS) of 1998, have confirmed that the Goal in type II Diabetes must also be normalization or near normalization of the blood glucose level in order to decrease associated complications.

Idea of writing this book is to give information to all Diabetic patients about the disease and its complications in a simple language so that they can understand these and can lead normal life.

Dr. A.K. Jhingan
Director
Delhi Diabetic Research Centre

J-136, Rajouri Garden,
New Delhi
Phones : 25419777, 25163623

Acknowledgements

More than 13,600 Diabetic patients who are registered with DDRC and attend this clinic regularly and provide information which is utilized in the interest of developing newer and better modes of treatment.

Experiences of many Physicians and Diabetic Educators has helped me to prepare this book.

I would like to thank the Management of Physicians of DDRC, who have helped me in great extent in preparing 3rd edition of this book.

I am also thankful to the Management and Staff of State Bank of India, who have helped me in organizing these Diabetes detection and education camps.

Pharmaceutical companies like NOVO-NORDISK (INDIA) PVT. LIMITED, BOEHRINGER MANNHEIM, HOECHST AND ELI LILLY RANBAXY LIMITED, SERDIA AND B.D. have also helped in providing educational materials in organising Diabetes detection and education camps.

My wife Dr. Kamalesh and children Kavita and Ram Mohan need special mention as without their cooperation this book would not have been completed.

In the end my special thanks to member and staff of Concept Publishing Company who helped me to accomplish the task of completing this 3rd edition of this book.

Dr. A.K. Jhingan

Contents

Diabetes Mellitus

Diabetes Mellitus is a word derived from Greek word Diabetos which means Siphon, Mellitus means Sweet, i.e. "flowing of sweet liquid."

There is mention of this disease by Ayurvedic physician Susruta in Ayurveda in about 400 B.C. and he had described it as "Honeyed urine." Charak, another physician of that time was also well aware of this disease (A.D.G.) A.D.

At present there are about 150 million people in the world with diabetes and many more may not be aware of their problem. It is expected that by the year 2000 this number would be around 176 million. Many more may not be aware about this disease and they may come to know only while undergoing tests for some problem or when they develop some complication of this disease.

What is Diabetes?

Main items of food are carbohydrates, proteins, fats, vitamins, minerals and water. Whatever food we take, from stomach it goes to small intestine then to large intestine. Many enzymes which come from stomach, gall bladder, liver, small intestine and pancreasomet gland, mix with food to make it more digestible. Carbohydrates are converted into glucose which gets into the blood stream and ultimately to cells of body to provide energy. This process of absorption of glucose from intestines and to enter into the cells of body is regulated through the "hoemone" called Insulin, secreted by gland called 'Pancreas'. In the deficiency of this hormone (Insulin), glucose will not enter into the cells and would remain in blood stream. Thus Blood Sugar will remain high and this sugar will pass in urine. As cells do not get sugar, there will be no energy. Person would feel weak and this will result in weight loss.

Normal Blood Sugar Level

Normal fasting Blood Sugar should be between 60 mg to 110 mg per 100ml of Blood. Blood Sugar 2 hours after food should be less than 140mg/ 100ml of Blood. When Blood Sugar is above this level it means person is suffering from Diabetes.

When the Blood Sugar is persistently high it circulates through kidney and other organs of body as it is not entering the cells.

Kidney cannot cope with this increased level of glucose and glucose escapes into the urine. Glucose will not appear in the urine until and unless Blood Sugar is above 180mg/100ml of Blood.

When there is absolute deficiency of Insulin fats also escape from fat cells and this fat is converted into Ketones, an acidic substance, by then more and more Ketones are released by liver into blood circulation it leads to *Ketoacidosis*. Ketones appear in urine. Ketones are not present in urine of a normal person.

So you have read above about Insulin Hormone which is very essential for the entry of glucose into cells and in the absence of this Hormone Blood Sugar level rises, sugar appear in urine and in the severe deficiency of this Hormone, i.e. insulin ketones also appear in urine which is a dangerous stage.

Insulin is secreted from Beta Cells of Pancrease gland located in the abdomen. How and why it stops functioning it is not known.

There are many factors which may be responsible for this stage which are discussed below.

Heredity

You must have observed that this disease runs in family. Many members of one family are suffering from diabetes. From parents, through genes it is transmitted to children, children will have defect in the Beta Cells which produce Insulin and so they become prone to develop diabetes.

This is commonly seen in Type II diabetes as compared to Type I diabetes.

Chances of Developing Diabetes

There are 25 to 30% chances of developing diabetes in the children of Type II diabetic patients.

If both parents are Type II diabetic then chances are 75%.

(HLA Antigens are associated with type I diabetes, further study is going on.)

Viruses. There are some studies which say that children who suffered from various virus diseases in childhood develop diabetes.

Obseity (Motapa). Obesity certainly predispose the individual to Diabetes specially Type II.

It is said that if person is 30 to 40% over weight than the weight indicated in standard height and weight tables, efficacy of Insulin is decreased by 30 to 40%.

There is insulin resistance. Although these patients are having high levels of insulin in the blood yet their Blood Sugar levels are high.

Diet

It has been observed that people who eat more refined sugars and diet rich in carbohydrate are prone to develop Diabetes. Incidence of Diabetes is higher in Indians who have migrated to U.K. or USA than the local inhabitants. The reason is that they might be having genetic predisposition and by consuming more sugar and carbohydrates in diet, they become obese, which itself is a risk factor for developing diabetes.

Diet rich in fibre reduces the incidence of Diabetes.

Drugs

Many drugs predispose Diabetes. Drugs like steroids used for Allergy and Asthma problems can aggravate diabetes.

Diuretics

Drugs which increase urine flow are used for high Blood pressure can also aggravate diabetes. These drugs lower Postassium which interfere with Insulin release thereby causing high Blood Sugar.

Oral contraceptives also increase Blood Sugar levels.

Lifestyle

Persons who are having borderline diabetesm i.e. Diabetes is yet not diagnosed when exposed to stress in life will manifest full-fledged disease. Sometimes, when you are undergoing investigation for some other disease like Chronic Diarrhoea, longstanding infection or extreme weakness, tests will reveal that you are having high Blood Sugar levels.

Types of Diabetes Mellitus

Types of Diabetes depends upon the status of Insulin Hormone in the body. They are Type I or Type II.

A. Type I or IDDM

If there is no Insulin or very less amount of Insulin then one has to be given Insulin injections regularly and this is called as 'Insulin Dependent Diabetes Mellitus' or IDDM or Type I Diabetes. These patients are young with rapid onset. If Insulin injections are not given to them they develop ketones in urine — and develops *Ketoacidosis* and *coma*. They can lead normal life with regular injections of Insulin. It usually manifest from the age of 4-5 years and these children would require daily Injections of Insulin to survive.

B. Type II DM or NIDDM

In these patients either there is deficiency of Insulin or resistance to the normal insulin action in the body. Usually there is family history of Diabetes in these patients. This is again of two types:

(a) Obese NIDDM — those who are over weight
(b) Non-Obese NIDPM

This type of Diabetes is usually seen in the people who are above the age of 40, it is also called as 'Maturity onset Diabetes'. More than 2/3rd of all Diabetic patients are suffering from Type II Diabetes. In this group of patients Diabetes can be controlled by Diet Restriction, Regular Exercise, and Oral Hypoglycaemic Agents, i.e. Tablets. Insulin injections are usually not required, initially, but later they may also require Insulin injection.

Symptoms of Diabetes

One of the most important symptoms of Diabetes is:
* Extreme weakness or lethargy.

Common Symptoms of Diabetes

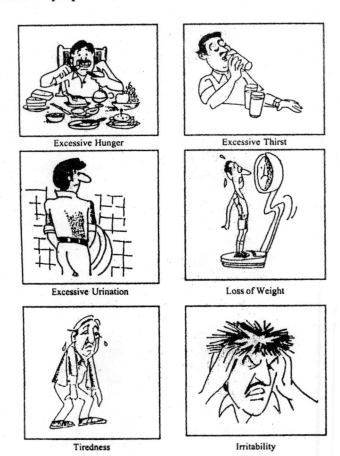

Excessive Hunger

Excessive Thirst

Excessive Urination

Loss of Weight

Tiredness

Irritability

Other symptoms are:

* Excessive Appetite.
* Excessive thirst (desire to take more and more water).
* Excessive urination.
* Loss of weight.
* Itching all over body and itching around private parts. Excessive itching around glands and penis in males and around vagina in females.
* Deterioration in vision with frequent changing of glasses.
* Leg cramps—Pain in legs.
* Burning, in both feet and numbness.
* Delayed healing of wound or some infection in the body.

Problems which Diabetics Encounter more often than General Public

* Heart Attacks (Specially at Young Age)
* Strokes, Paralytic Attacks
* Gangrene of Foot—Leading to Amputation of Foot or Toe
* Repeated Attacks of Infections or Boils
* Rapid Deterioration of Vision and Blindness
* Sexual Problems
* Kidney Disease and Need for dialysis or Renal Transplant.
* Giddiness.
* Eyes-blurring of vision or double vision called Diplopia are common eye symptoms in diabetic patients.

There had been increase in the number of Diabetic patients. Reasons behind this increase are:

* Change in lifestyle.
* Change in food habits.
* Awareness about the disease and symptoms. Patients come forward for blood tests and other investigations for the diagnosis of Diabetes.

Testing of Sugar

Various Diabetes detection and education programmes have changed the thinking of general population. Now they believe that early diagnosis of Diabetes and its control can make their life comfortable, free from the complications of Diabetes. There are various methods to diagnose Diabetes. These are:

* Urine Examination for sugar.
* Blood test for glucose.

Urine Examination

Urine can be tested for glucose at home or in laboratory by stick method or by Benedicts test.

Test by Glucostrips

This is simple procedure, various companies make strips. There is a chemical at the end of strip which when comes in contact with urine sugar/glucose changes its colour. One can read and compare the colours with the colours displayed at strip bottle.

How to do it

1. Collect urine in small container an dip the strip in it for a few seconds or one can dip the strip in stream while passing urine.

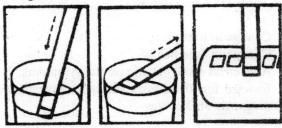

2. Shake and clean the strip to remove the excess amount of urine on it.
3. After one minute compare the colour of strip with the colours depicted at bottle.

Results

From the strip it will become clear whether one is having sugar or not. +, ++, ++++ of sugar or 0.5%, 1%, 1.5% or 2%.
Depending upon the colour of strip from

* Blue
* Dark Green
* Yellow-Green
* Brown
* Orange.

It is not essential that all Diabetic patients will pass sugar in urine. If Blood Sugar is not more than 180 mg, 100 ml of Blood Sugar will not appear in urine.

Excessive intake of Vita-C/Asprin or Aldomet tablets can give false results, i.e. if person is taking the above medicines his urine may not reveal correct picture.

With Benedict Test

Urine is heated with Benedict solution and change in colour is observed. Depending upon the colour of mixture — If it is Blue, Dark Green, Yellow Green, Orange. Strips for ketone are also available, IDDM patients urine should be tested for Ketones in urine.

Urine testing for sugar can be done 3-4 times a day in a patient who is using insulin to monitor the dose of Insulin.

Blood Sugar Estimation

For Blood Sugar estimation now-a-days there are computerised equipment available which can give the results within few minutes.

Blood Sugar estimation can be done

    A. Fasting Blood Sugar
    B. Post Prandial
    C. Random

Fasting Blood Sugar is usually between

*   60 to 110mg%
*   Post Prandial (PP) means two hours after the meals, i.e. food, not two hours after 1st Blood samples were collected. This Blood Sugar should be below 140 mg%.

Random Blood Sugar means levels at any time of the day which should be below 160mg% in normal person.

Blood Sugar can be done by Gluconometer. It is an easy process require only drop of blood and results are know at the same time.

Blood Sugar (Self Analysis How Much Under Control)

	Empty Stomach (Fasting)	After 2 hours, of Food (PP)
Normal Level	110mg%	140mg%
Satisfactory Level	120mg%	160mg%
Uncontrolled	Above 140mg%	Above 200mg%

There are many types of Gluconometer available in the market at present and are easy to use.

We need strips which have pad at one end which reacts with blood and changes its colour which can be read by naked eye or by feeding strip into the Gluconometer which reveals Blood Sugar level.

Method

    1. Clean the finger and then press the Autoclix or prick the finger with needle.
    2. Massage the finger to bring big drop of blood on yellow pad, i.e. coloured portion of strip.

3. Keep this strip for one minute on a plane surface after drop of blood.
4. Take cotton and clean the blood from the strip in a one process. Don't rub the strip again and again. At this stage you have two options if you have gluconometer then insert the strip (coloured portion) facing you or you wait for one more minute if you don't have gluconometer and after one minute compare the colours with the colours which given on bottle you can read 200mg, 400mg or 500mg% or gluconometer will show the Blood glucose level on meter. If you have other gluconometer then you have to wait for the gluconometer to show 22 seconds and you will hear a beep and then soak the blood, feed the stick into gluconometer and at the end of 50 seconds you can read Blood sugar level.

Blood Sugar Estimation from Laboratory

By giving blood in laboratory you can be the report. Regular Blood Sugar testing is essential to know the result of treatment and one can adjust the does.

Blood Sugar test should be done twice, i.e. in fasting stage and 2 hours after food.

There is doubt in the mind of all diabetics that the blood sugar estimation by gluconometer is not reliable. It is not true, throughout the world these gluconometers are used. Usually there is difference of 10 to 15 mg in the reading of the gluconometer and the readings from outside, i.e. laboratory.

If there is doubt then one can undergo Glucose Tolerance Test.

Glucose Tolerance Test (G.T.T.)

In this test the person is given 75gm of glucose on the day of test and Blood samples are collected every 30 minutes of 2 hourly and then hourly. Now-a-days many labs don't insist upon taking many samples of blood. Blood glucose more than 200mg% one to two hour after glucose ingestion are diagnostic of Diabetes.

Precautions

The person who is undergoing G.T.T., should eat large amount of carbohydrate and should exercise regularly and should not be suffering from any serious disease.

1. Person should not eat anything 8 to 10 hours before test.
2. Person undergoing G.T.T., after giving Ist or IInd blood sample should not go for walking otherwise it will alter Blood Sugar levels.
3. He should not smoke during this period.

People who should undergo this test

1. Suspected cases of Diabetes.
2. Persons having Family History of Diabetes.
3. Obese person.
4. Persons suffering from tuberculosis or non-healing ulcers.
5. Family History of heart attacks in young age.
6. Persons whose Blood Sugar level rises during stress phases should undergo this test.

Glycosylated Haemoglobin—HbA$_{IC}$

Blood test which indicates Blood Sugar levels in a Diabetic patients over a period of last 2-3 months. Specially useful in Diabetes with pregnancy and it helps to give an idea about the efficacy of treatment. If one can afford one should undergo this test atleast once or twice in a year.

Normal levels are expressed in %. Normal levels are less than 6.4%. If it is persistently above 9% it indicates abnormally high Blood Sugar and need proper control.

HbA$_{IC}$ — Normal valure 5.2% - 6.4%

Reduction of HbA$_{IC}$ below 7% reduces incidence of complication. If the HbA$_{IC}$ levels are kept below or around 6.5% there are less chances of complications.

Summary About Tests for Diabetes

* One should regularly get his urine tested for sugar and keep records.
* If there is history of vomiting and loose motions get urine tested for Ketones because timely examination of Ketones in urine can prevent the person going into coma.
* At least once in a year urine should be tested for proteins in urine (even in small amount called microalbumin uria). Appearance of Albumin in urine indicates involvement of kidneys in diabetes and at this stage if Blood Sugar is kept under control further damage to kidney can be prevented.
* Each diabetic patient should have blood sugar test daily if he is on Insulin and once weekly if he is on tablets.

Self Monitoring

All Diabetics should learn to monitor their diabetes themselves by doing urine test and Blood glucose estimation. This is called as Home Blood Glucose Monitoring (HBGM). You can make diary and can write about Blood Sugar Levels which will indicate that your Diabetes is under control or not. H.B.G.M. is useful in following situations:

1. This is very important for Diabetic patients who are taking Insulin injections. By measuring Blood Sugar they can reduce or increase the Insulin dose and can prevent Hyper or Hypoglycemia.
2. Useful in those patients who are advised strict Diabetic control.
3. In Brittle Diabetics it is useful where Blood Sugar level fluctuates.
4. In Diabetic patients with kidney involvement.
5. Persons using Insulin pumps or 3-4 injections of Insulin daily.
6. It is very useful in patients of Diabetes with pregnancy.

What is Meant by Good Control

1. Normal blood sugar levels.
2. Weight — as near to ideal as possible.
3. Blood pressure should be normal.
4. Blood cholesterol and triglycerides within normal limits.
5. Glycosylated hemoglobin within normal limits.

Treatment of Diabetes Mellitus

Diabetics who know more about the disease, its complications and how to cope with it can live longer than those who are aware about it.

Diabetes is a disease which can be controlled by Diet, exercise, oral medications and Insulin. There is no short-cut as regard management of diabetes is concerned. Treatment plan has to be discussed with patient. He has to be informed about side effects of medicines and about complications of Diabetes which will develop if untreated. It requires patience by both patient as well as his or her relatives. Chances of complications can be significantly reduced if Blood Sugar is kept under control.

Diet

The most important thing you can do to balance your Blood Sugar is to eat the right food. You should follow a well balanced food plan. Each person requires different amount of calories per day depending upon weight, height and type of work the individual is doing. Food you eat consists of carbohydrate, protein, fat, vitamins, minerals, fibre and water. Each one gm of carbohydrate gives 4 calories, 1 gm of fat gives 9 calories and each 1 gm of protein gives 4 calories. Extra weight puts a strain on your system. Your body is less able to use Insulin, and it is difficult for your tablets to control your blood Sugar. Extra weight leads to poor control of Diabetes and may contribute to serious complications. Your doctor will help you to lose weight. Don't try to lose weight any faster than 0.5 kg per week.

Your Diet Contains

Carbohydrate which provides 50 to 60% energy. This is present in sugar, honey, jam, cereals, flour, bread, rice, and dairy products.

Protein: Is required for growth and provides 10 to 20% energy. Protein is present in milk, milk products, meat, nuts, eggs, cereals and pulses.

Fat: Fat provides 30% of energy. Fat consists of fatty acids, and glycerol.

A. *Fat Rich in Saturated Fatty Acids:* Animal fat (meat products), Dairy products (ghee, butter, cream), and coconut oil. Animal fat contains plenty of cholesterol.

B. *Mono Saturated Fats:* These are: olive oil, plam oil, ground nut oil.

C. *Fat Rich in Poly-Unsaturated Fatty Acids (PUFA):* These are, sun flower oil, safflower oil, soyabean oil, corn oil, cotton seed oil, fish oil, High temperature destroys the structure of above oils (PUFA). Hence deep frying should be avoided.

Fibre in Diet: Includes indigestible plant cell components present in diet. These are present in cereals, pulses, vegetables, fruits and nuts.

Fibre is of two types.

One: Which is present in skin, and husks of fruits. It helps in preventing constipation as it has laxative effect.

Other type: It holds water and form gel. Isafgol is an important source, other sources are fenu greek, oats, barley, plums, raisins beans and carrots.

Fibre in diet helps in

1. Controlling diabetes by preventing excessive rise in blood glucose after meals.
2. Helps in decreasing blood cholesterol and triglycerides so less chances of getting heart attack.
3. Helps in reducing weight: Becomes bulky and gives feeling of fullness thereby lowers appetite and calorie intake.

How Much Calories are Needed

If you are over weight	20 cal/kg/day
If you are ideal weight	30 cal/kg/day
If you are under weight	40 cal/kg/day

Weight is calculated as per the height and body frame tables.
The basic principles behind creating high quality Health Foods are:

1. Add alteast 2% dietary fibres to all preparations.
2. Use only those ingredients which are rich in fibres, vitamins, minerals and flavonoids, such as, whole grains, vegetables/fruits.
3. Use ingredients which are rich in EFAs, sterols and antioxidant Vitamin E, like wheat germs, soyabean, sesame and almond/apricot.
4. Keep density of foods light and make these balanced, i.e. proper ratio of proteins, carbohydrates, fibres and fats.

Artificial/Alternate Sweeteners—Saccharine

Saccharine should be added after cooking not before cooking. Saccharine should be avoided in pregnancy. Use should be restricted to a maximum of 7 tablets.

Aspartame - 1 packet contains 35 gm aspartame.

Available as Sweeter, sugar free, equal etc. All above sweeters should be avoided in pregnancy and in children.

Alcohol - One has not to give up alcohol because he is diabetic.

You should keep the use within sensible limits—(one or two drinks, i.e. 30-45ml of alcohol). Alcohol provides empty calories. It can interfere with tablets you take for diabetes control and may cause very low Blood Sugar.

Fruits

Which fruits and vegetables can be taken—

* Fruits are good low calorie snack with valuable fibre, vitamins and minerals. Fruit juices may be taken in small quantity, if at all.
* Salad vegetables are filling and also valuable sources of vitamins, minerals and fibre.
* Pulses vegetables, e.g. peas, beans and lentils have a beneficial effect on blood glucose and lipid levels and

are a good source of Protein with soluble fibre.
* Encourage fruit and vegetable as a part of overall healthy eating.

Fats

* Fats are Major Source of Energy and to cut down on fat intake is important especially if weight reduction is required.
* Hidden source of fats—Biscuits, fatty meals, pies, pastry, full fat dairy products, should be avoided.

Proteins

* Avoid excessive Proteins in long standing diabetes if patient is passing protein in urine. Proteins are restricted in diet.
* Pulses — Peas, beans, lentils are high in soluble fibre and Iron.
* Fish can be taken — 2-3 times in a week.

Which Sweeteners

Not Honey As It Equates With Sugar

Non-nutritive sweetners, e.g., Saccharine, Aspartame are suitable especially if weight is a problem.

Avoid Sorbitol and Fructose.

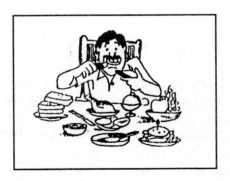

Ghee or Refined Vegetable Oil

There has been a sudden and sharp rise in prevalence of many diseases specially heart disease, kidney disease and Diabetes. It is because, we have deviated from our traditional low fat diet and have adopted fast food culture.

This fast, fatty, fried, refined, processed and preserved food has ill-balanced high fat content. It is deficit in an important essential fatty acid (n:3fat) which is found in green leafy vegetables, mustard oil and seeds, fish oil, flax seed, and *methy*. This type of food contains n:6 fatty acids and high content of unsaturated fats.

People have been using ghee, butter and milk and yet they were having good health. Since the case of these vegetable redefined oils, there has been sharp increase in use of diabetes and heart diseases. Intake of storage fat and refined vegetable oils lead to weight gain and obesity. These adverse effect can be attributed to high content of Polyunsaturated n:6 fat contained in these animal fats and vegetable oils. Cholesterol in ghee and milk is limited in quantity. Indians consuming typical Indian diet do not get even the half the required quantity of cholesterol. One can use. 2-3 teaspoon full of Ghee per person per day or 1/2 kg per month. Don't fry the items in Ghee. In India we have used these for centuries without any harm. The reason was people were using ghee, milk or butter and were doing regular exercise. Life was not sedentary as it is today. You can use Desi Ghee, milk and butter but should do regular exercise for at lease 30 minutes a day.

Dietitian

Every Diabetic Should consult Dietitian who is expert in food and nutrition. Dietitian can help you to find out your food needs based on your weight, lifestyle and the type of treatment you are taking.

Fats in Blood

Fats include Cholesterol and Triglycerides. Our body make cholesterol and triglycerides. We can also get them from animal foods.

Cholesterol is used by body for making cell walls and certain vitamins and minerals. Triglyceride is stored fat, and gives you energy reserves. Triglycerdes keep you warm and protect the body organs.

Triglycerides and cholesterol are carried in Blood by Lipoproteins.

1. ULDL: Carries cholesterol and triglycerides and other fats in fat tissues.
2. Low-Density Lipoprotein (L.D.L.): L.D.L. carries cholesterol to parts of the body that need it. L.D.L. can stick to blood vessel walls. Cholesterol on Blood vessel wall leads to occlusion and thus coronary Artery Disease. The less L.D.L. in your Blood, the better.
3. High Density Lipoprotein (H.D.L.) : It carries cholesterol away from the blood vessel walls to the liver. Liver breaks the cholesterol down and sends it out of the body. The more H.D.L. in your blood, the better.

Diabetic patients have high blood fats and these high levels make them prone to develop heart disease, heart-attack, and stroke.

What should be your Blood fat Levels
* Total Cholesterol LESS THAN 180 Mg/dl
* L.D.L. Cholesterol LESS THAN 100 Mg/dl
* H.D.L Cholesterol MORE THAN women >55Mg/dl, Men > 45 Mg/dl
* Triglycerides LESS THAN 150 Mg/dl

How to Improve Your Blood fat Levels

* Control Your Blood Sugar Levels.
* If you are over-weight, then lose few kilograms. Losing weight raises your good H.D.L. Cholesterol.
* More fat you eat, the more V.L.D.L. the liver makes More V.L.D.L. Means Bad L.D.L. Cholesterol.
* Replace saturated fats (Desi Ghee and Butter) with unsaturated fats (Vegetable oils). Saturated fats raise your L.D.L. and unsaturated fats lower them.
* Avoid foods which have high Cholesterol.
* Eat foods, high in fiber. Beans, peas, fresh fruits are rich in fiber.
* Aerobic exercises such as brisk walk, jogging, and swimming, raise your good H.D.L. Cholesterol.
* Smoking lowers good H.D.L. Cholesterol. So quit or cut down.

Have your Lipid profile tested at least once a year.

Diabetes and High Blood Pressure

People with Diabetes are more likely to have high blood pressure than non-diabetics. High blood pressure is a Risk factor for having a heart attack, or stroke and may cause or worsen kidney disease and retinopathy (eye disease).

Blood pressure is the force of your blood as it travels through your blood vessels. The higher your blood pressure, the more force on your blood vessels and this can weaken and damage blood vessels and finally damages organs and nerves.

Symptoms

High Blood Pressure (Hypertension) leads to
- Weakness, Headache,
- Fatigue, Tiredness
- Irritability

On each visit to your doctor you must get your blood pressure checked.

It is reported as systolic and diastolic Blood pressure. Systolic Blood Pressure is the force of your blood when your heart contracts. Diastolic pressure is the force of your blood when heart relaxes.

Blood pressure is written as 130/80 mm of Hg

130 is Systolic Blood pressure. 80 is Diastolic Pressure. It is measured as m.m./hg.

Target Blood Pressure

In adults with Diabetes

* Normal less than 130/80
* Mild hypertension 130/80 to 140/90
* Moderae Hypertension 140/90 to 160/100
* Severe Hypertension 160/100 and above

Many people still think Blood pressure for different age groups is different. They calculate Blood Pressure as age +100.

This is wrong. For all adults blood pressure should be less than 130/80.

In patients with Type I Diabetes, High Blood Pressure is often caused by underlying diabetic kidney disease.

In Type II Diabetic patients it is present in more than 50% of cases at the time of diagnosis, as a part of diabetic metabolic disorder.

Aggressive blood pressure control reduces the vascular complications of diabetes.

To Lower Your Blood Pressure

1. *Reduce excess weight* :- Loosing few kg weight can bring your blood pressure to normal. Best way to lose weight is to follow a weight-loss diet and an exercise programme.

2. *Stop Smoking* :- Smoking plays important role in causing

blood pressure by damaging blood vessls. Stopping smoking can help not only in lowering the risk of Hypertension related death but also reduces the number of blood pressure controlling medicines.

3. *Reduce Alcohol Intake*:- More than 60ml intake of alcohol everyday may cause high blood pressure. 30ml alcohol twice or three times a week may be taken if one cannot live without it.

4. *Eat less salt* :- Reducing the amount of salt may be enough to lower your blood pressure.

5. *Reduce stress* :- Stress may increase your blood pressure. During stress blood vessels constrict and Heart has to work hard.

If blood pressure does not come down then your doctor may put you on drugs to lower your blood pressure.

Lifestyle

The basic concept of a healthy lifestyle is:

* Maintain your body weight according to your age and height by controlling calories intake.
* Regular exercise is the only key to keep Blood Sugar and Blood Pressure under control only with weight.
* Discard "junk foods" which are loaded with saturated fats and/or sugar (all deep fried food, chocolates, ice creams, artificial drinks).
* Discard alcohol and tobacco and cut down on tea/coffee.
* Adopt natural foods, vegetables, fruits, cereals, legumes and nuts and only scientifically processed health foods (always look for the labels).
* Cut down the size of your meals and increase the frequency.
* Do not restrict your diet to a few selected food — *variety is the key.*

Exercise

Importance of Exercise is mentioned in all ancient books and Ayurveda. Physicians like Shushrata and Charak have mentioned the benefits of exercise especially in Diabetic patients.

According to them they have advised horse riding, long brisk walks and wrestling for obese diabetic patients. Participation in above sports and all other sports reduces blood sugar levels.

Every person should consult his physician before joining any exercise programme. Exercise programme is different for each individual and it depends upon many factors like age of patient and associated high blood pressure and other problems. If Physician advises you to undergo some investigations like E.C.G. etc., then you must undergo these investigations.

Exercise should be performed five days in a week, 40-45 minutes each day one should start exercise gradually and increase it slowly.

Certain points to remember—

* Exercise should be performed on an empty stomach.
* One should wear loose and comfortable clothes (dress).
* One should avoid lifting of heavy weights.
* Avoid exercise in extreme hot or cold climate.

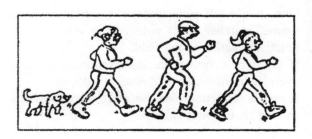

Precautions for Exercise

Before starting an exercise programme, certain factors to be kept in mind:

* If one is over 40 years of age.
* If one has never participated in strenuous physical activity since younger days.
* If one is over weight.
* If one is a heavy smoker.
* If one has high blood pressure or is suffering from angina.

Evaluation by a physician and complete health checkup including E.C.G. are essential prior to undertaking any exercise programme for the above mentioned people. Persons with diabetic foot and peripheral vascular disease, should avoid running, and choose cycling or swimming for exercise.

In the presence of retinal involvement (retinopathy), diabetics should avoid exercise associated with increased abdominal pressure or sudden acceleration or trauma to head and lifting of weight. In the presence of hypertension, avoid heavy weight lifting and choose exercise that involve lower limbs, i.e.walking.

One should observe the following precautions during exercise:

* Start with warm up exercises.
* One should not exercise straight after eating.
* Exercise should not be done under extremes of temperature.
* It is unwise to exercise if one has some infection or common cold.
* One should not participate in competitive programmes (game, matches, etc.) unless fully trained or has been practising earlier in the field.
* If chest pain occurs during exercise, one should stop exercise immediately and consult a doctor.
* If one is restarting exercise after a break of 2 weeks or so, one should start slowly.

Advantage of Exercise

Regular Exercise prevents risk factors for heart attack and high blood pressure.

* Fat and cholesterol levels fall with regular exercise.
* It gives you feeling of well being.
* Utilisation of calories helps to control weight.
* Reduces weight.
* Helps in controlling blood sugar.

Precautions before Exercise

If you have heart or joint problems or are very overweight or have never exercised much before, it is particularly important that you talk to your doctor. If you develop chest or leg pains during exercise it is important to stop exercising and tell your doctor.

* Walk upstairs instead of taking a lift.
* Don't sit down when you are waiting for bus or train. But stroll about instead.
* Play more actively with your children or grandchildren.
* Take your dog for longer walks.
* Wear comfortable, well-fitting shoes and socks for exercising.
* Cool down at the end of the session by gradually decreasing your level of exercise over 5-10 minutes.

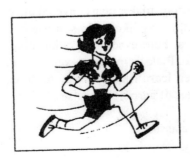

What Type? How to Achieve Target? What Precautions?

Aerobic exercises are ones that use your heart, lungs, arms, and legs. By working these parts of your body, you can improve your blood flow, reduce your risk of heart disease, and lower your blood pressure. You can also lower your LDL cholesterol (bad cholestrol) and triglycerides and raise your HDL cholesterol (the good cholestrol).

When you do aerobic exercises, you breathe harder and your heart beats faster. This builds your endurance and increases your energy. You may find that aerobic exercises help you sleep better, make you feel less stressed, balances your emotions, and improves your sense of well-being.

Aerobic exercise is not only good for your heart but is also good for your diabeties. Aerobic exercise makes your Insulin work harder and faster, reduces your body fat, and helps you lose weight. If you don't exercise already, your doctor may advise you to start.

What to do Before you Start

Check with your doctor before you start any exercise. Your doctor may want some tests to see how your heart, blood vessels, eyes, feet, and nerves are doing. Your blood pressure, blood fat levels, glycohemoglobin levels, and body fat might also be checked. Your doctor or nurse can tell you how to adjust your diabetes-care plan for exercise.

What Aerobic Exercises to do

Some exercises may make heart, eye, feet, or nerve problems worse. Your doctor may like to do some test to check your heart and blood vessels, before advising what kinds of exercises are safe for you to do. Pick from these exercises a few you think you might enjoy. Then learn the right way to do each exercise. Here are some examples of aerobic exercises:

* Aerobic classes
* Bicycling

* Dancing
* Jogging
* Jumping rope
* Rowing
* Running
* Skating (roller, ice, in-line)
* Skiing (downhill, cross-country)
* Stair climbing
* Swimming
* Walking

How Long and How Often to Exercise

If you are just starting to exercise after a long time of little or no activity, go for 5 minutes. Build up to short bouts of exercise that add up to at least 30 minutes a day. For example, you might try brisk walking or stair climbing for 10 minutes three times a day or for 15 minutes twice a day.

Exercising for less than 15 minutes a day is not likely to improve your health. Gradually build up to 20 to 60 minutes of continuous aerobic exercise three to five times a week. The 20 to 60 minutes of aerobic exercise does not include your warm-up and cooldown.

A warm-up will slowly raise your heart rate, warm your muscles, and help prevent injuries. A cooldown will lower your heart rate and slow your breathing. Warm up for 5 to 10 minutes before aerobic exercise, and cooldown for 5 to 10 minutes after aerobic exercise. As a warm-up or a cool down, you could gently stretch, walk, or slowly bicycle.

How Hard to Exercise

Your doctor, nurse, or exercise specialist can tell you how hard to exercise by giving you a number. The number is a percentage. It may be as low as 40 per cent or as high as 70 per cent. It is a percentage of your capacity for exercise (your maximum aerobic capacity). There are a few ways to figure out your maximum aerobic capacity. Here's one easy way.

Subtract your age from 220. The answer is your maximum heart rate. For example, if you are 40, your maximum heart rate is 180. To exercise at 60 per cent of your maximum aerobic capacity, keep your pulse at 108 beats per minute (180 × 60% = 108). A nurse can show you how to take your pulse.

When to Exercise

A good time to exercise is 1 to 3 hours after you finish a meal or snack. The food you have eaten will help keep your blood glucose level from falling too low.

Do not Exercise when

* Your blood glucose level is over 300mg/dl.
* Your insulin or diabetes pills are peaking.
* You have ketones in your urine.
* You have numbness, tingling, or pain in your feet or legs.
* You are short or breath.
* You are ill.
* You have a serious injury.
* You feel dizzy.
* You have pain/tightness in your chest, neck, shoulders, or jaw.
* You have blurred sight of blind spots.

Role of Yoga

There are various schools of thought and according to them various yogic exercises are good for controlling Blood Sugar levels. Some of the *ASANAS* are specially useful for controlling Diabetes.

Dangers of Exercise (Without medical supervision)

Before planning for Exercise one should consult Doctor to evaluate his cardiac status. If person is having underlying heart disease and he/she starts strenuous exercise it might precipitate fresh attack of angina or heart attack and may even cause death. In old age arthritis also restricts the movements of joints and can cause stiffness in joints.

Yoga has become popular all over world. System of Yoga was developed by great *yogis* and *saints* thousands of years ago. It teaches discipline and keeps the body physically fit.

One can learn the art of yoga by regular practice. Initially it would be difficult to assume the correct posture but gradually one can learn. Before trying yoga; please consult your doctor.

Following yogic exercises are useful for diabetic patients. Although there are many asanas but I have selected a few which can be done easily without much difficulty.

1. Ardhnav Asana

It helps to activate functioning of gall bladder, kidneys and pancrease.

2. Dhanur Asana

It activates all glands of body specially Pancrease and helps in release of Insulin hormone.

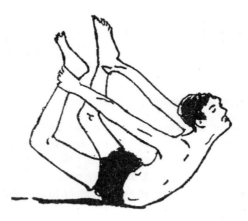

3. Janusshirsh Asana

This asana helps in improving the functioning of Liver and Pancrease.

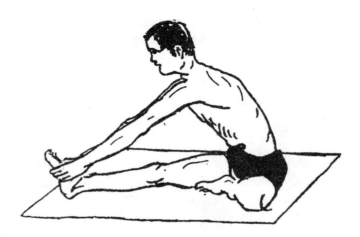

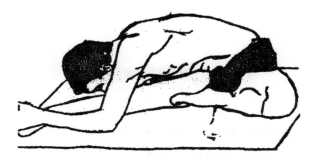

4. Ardhmatsyendra Asana

This asana is specially useful for diabetics and it stimulates the functioning of Pancrease gland.

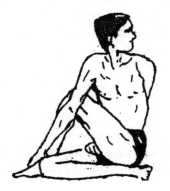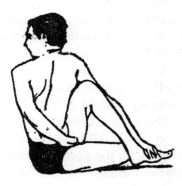

Precautions

* In persons who are having Retinal involvement (Eye involvement) strenuous exercise may cause Retinal detachment and sudden blindness.
* Take care of your food before and after exercise and inspect for any vesicles, cuts or any change in colour of nails.
* One should keep sugar with one self as suddenly Blood Sugar may fall during exercise and intake of sugar will prevent hypoglycemia (low blood sugar).

Drug Treatment

Oral Hypoglycemic Agens (OHA)/Tablets

If by regular exercise and with proper food control Blood Sugar is not under control then patient is advised to take medicines for lowering Blood Sugar.

Diabetes is chronic problem and one had to take medicines for a longer time along with diet control and exercise.

It the Random blood sugar level is persistently above 250mg% in spite of good diet control and regular exercise your doctor will advise you to take medicines these are tablets belonging to two different groups Sulfonyl Urea and Bigunides.

All the medicines are given in low doses initially and patients are advised to take these medicines before meals or after meals—depending upon the medicine.

There are different indications for these medicines so each patient should follow doctor's advise and should not change these tablets as per the advise of other patient. One should avoid taking medicines along with alcohol as sometimes there can be severe adverse effects of it.

* One should avoid taking extra dose of tablets with extra food or ice cream.
* One should avoid using these medicines if doctor has recommended the use of Insulin. As intake of these medicines in cases of kidney failure, liver diseases, heart diseases and chronic respiratory diseases may be harmful and dangerous.
* Different group of persons are advised different medicines by doctors, like fat and obese persons will be advised to take 2nd group of medicines, like Glyciphage or Glycomet

D.B.I. Capsule etc., so one should avoid changing medicines according to his will.

Main side effect of all these medicines is hypoglycemia, other side effect are itching all over body, Nausea, vomiting, giddiness, distension of adomen, constipation or diarrhoea.

Use of pain kills along with these drugs increases effects of these medicines.

Who are the persons who will need these tablets?

1. Persons with NIDDM or Maturity onset diabetes, i.e. above the age of 40 years.
2. Whose requirement for Insulin is less.
3. Whose diabetes is of short duration.
4. Use of these medicines along with Insulin, in adult patients.
5. Should not be given to children (IDDM) with Diabetes.

Points to Remember

*   *All tablets are not alike.* In one person tablet may be more effective while it may not be helpful to other. So don't change your medicines on other's advice.
*   For each patient different tablets are prescribed depending upon the weight, and nature of job. *So don't stop your tablets and change them without your Doctor's advice.*
*   Don't take *tablets with alcohol.*
*   If you have missed one dose don't take extra dose at one time.
*   Diabetic children should not be given tablets.
*   Pregnant ladies should not be given tablets if they are diabetic.
*   Tablets should be taken 1/2 an hour before breakfast and dinner.

List of Tablets Which are Available for Diabetes Control

Name	Strength of Available Tablet
Diabenese	100mg and 250 mg. Tablet
Restinon	500mg. Tablet
Daonil	2.5mg. and 5mg. Tablet
Euglucon	2.5 mg. and 5mg. Tablet
Etanase	5mg. Tablet
Glynase	5mg. Tablet
Dimicron	20mg. Tablet
Glizide	20mg. Tablet
Diabend	20mg. Tablet
Glycomet	500mg. Tablet
Glyciphage	500mg. Tablet
Diphage	500mg. Tablet
D.B.I.	25mg Capsule
DBI-TD	50mg. Capsule

These medicines should not be given to—

* Those who are undergoing major surgery like Coronary By-pass Surgery.
* Those suffering from severe infections.
* Patients with kidney failure.

In all above cases patients are advised to take Insulin and once recovery takes place then one can switch on to oral medicines as per advice of Doctor.

Switch over to Insulin

If with diet control, exercise and full dosage of these medicines, Blood Sugar is not under control, i.e. above 200mg% then your Doctor will advise you to use Insulin injections to control diabetes.

* 10-15 years after using these tablets the efficacy of these medicines is decreased this is called secondary failure to these agents and such patients are advised to take Insulin.

WHAT YOU SHOULD KNOW ABOUT TABLETS

When Oral Hypoglycemic Agents (OHA) Tablets Fail

"Oral hypoglycemic agents have, in most patients, only a temporary effect." And many times after taking these tablets for many years there is no effect.

Primary Failure

"Approximately 30% of Type II diabetics fail to respond to oral hypoglycemic agents singly or in combinations even at presentation."

Secondary Failure

"About 5 to 10% of patients per year who respond initially to a sulfonylurea tablets, e.g. Daonil, Glynase, Euglucon etc., become secondary failures, as defined by unacceptable levels of hyperglycemia." They will not respond to these medicines and their Blood Sugar would remain high.

Changing Oral Agents does not improve Secondary Failure

"Patients who fail maximal doses first generation sulfonylurea should not be expected to respond to second-generation oral agent and should be changed to Insulin." One should avoid changing tablets from one brand to other as there will not be of any benefit at this stage.

NEWER ANTIDIABETIC MEDICINES

Useful in Controlling Post Prandial Hyperglycemia (High Blood Sugar levels after meals)

The main challenge of controlling diabetes is to achieve near normal Blood Sugar levels. For the same several classes of new oral medicines are now available among these are Alpha-glucosidase inhibitors like Acarbose, short acting insulinotropic agents rapid-acting insulin analogues and other agents.

Alpha-Glucosidase Inhibitors

ACARBOSE (Glucobay) delays the digestion of complex carbohydrates by competitively inhibiting intestinal Alpha-glucosidase. By delaying the digestion and prolonging the intestinal absorption of dietary carbohydrates, these agents diminish Post Prandial hyperglycemia?

Patients should take their dose of Glucobay etc. with the first bite of each meal. Side effect of this medicine is flatulence and loose stools.

Glitazones

These are insulin sensitisers. They act by blocking Peroxisome Proliferator receptor (PPAR) at adipose tissue. This adipogenic effect of PPAR contributes to insulin sensitisation. They diminish fatty acid uptake by muscles, thus improving Insulin resistance. Drugs available in market belong to:

    (a) Rosiglitazone (Rezult, Rosicon, Reglit etc.)
    (b) Pioglitazoe (Pioglet, Pioglae, Pioz etc.)

These drugs also decrease triglycerides and increase good cholesterol, i.e. HDL.

Repaglinide

It acts by stimulating insulin secretion. This drug is given three times daily 15 minutes before each meal. Because of its rapid onset drug is useful in controlling Post Prandial hyperglycemia.

Rapid Acting Insulin

Rapid Acting Insulin analogues are specially useful in controlling Post Prandial hyperglycemia. It is safe and effective in both Type I and Type II diabetes. Available as Humalog.

Insulin

Before the invention of Insulin it was difficult for Diabetic patients to survive beyond the age of 20 years. Now there are patients who are using Insulin from the last 30 to 40 years and leading normal life.

Insulin was invented in 1926 by Dr. Fredrik Banting and Dr. Charles West, since then many changes have taken place in the structure and potency. Today various types of Insulin are available for diabetic patients.

Insulin is hormone secreated by the pancrease.

There are three sources of *Insulin% Pork Insulin— Porcine Insulin, Beef Insulin, Bovine Insulin, Human Insulin.*

Now-a-days purified Insulin are also available.

Insulin are of two types

* Plane—colourless—Short Acting
* NPH or Lente—Milky colour—long Acting

Which patients need Insulin:

1. All patients of IDDM or Type I Diabetes (Insulin Dependent Diabetes patients).
2. Patients of NIDDM or Type II Diabetes (Non-Insulin Dependent Diabetes) who develop secondary drug failure to oral agents. In all such cases insulin is given for short period.
3. Pregnant diabetic mothers.
4. Diabetic patients who are undergoing major surgery like Coronary By-Pass Surgery, or Eye Surgery or other major surgery.
5. Patients who develop Kidney failure.

List of Insulins available

Different Insulin preparations are available depending upon the duration of action.

Fast Acting Insulins—which have short duration of Action
* Plane Insulin
* Actrapid Insulin
* Hum Insulin-R
* Insuman Rapid, etc.

Long Acting Insulins—which have longer duration of action
* Iletin-L
* Lentard
* Hum Insulin-L
* N.P.H. Insulin
* Insulintard
* Iletin-N
* Hum Insulin-N
* Hum Insulin Mixtard 30/70, 50/50
* Insuman 25/75, 50/50
* Mixtard Penfil
* Monotard, etc.

Even with Insulin injection one should follow strict diet control and regular Exercise Schedule.

Some Insulins are short acting, their effect starts immediately so one should take along with food. Other types of Insulins are intermediate or long acting, their action starts within 2-4 hours and lasts from 12 to 18 hours.

Types of Insulin available in India

Insulin injections are made as 40 units or/100units/ml depending upon the type of Insulin.

One should be careful while filling the syringe regarding the dose of Insulin and should consult Physician about adjusting the dose.

Insulin syringes are made up of plastic material one can use the same syringe 3 to 4 times. Insulin syringes can be kept in refrigerator after using it.

Your Doctor will advise you to take one injection or two injections or more depending upon the type of Diabetes and other associated conditions.

Oral drugs are also given along with Insulin in some cases for better control of Diabetes and weight.

Complications of Insulin Injections

1. Hypoglycemia (Low Blood Sugar).
2. Atrophy or abcess at the site of injection.
3. Itching at the site of injection.

These complications can be avoided by proper dosage of Insulin. Taking Insulin injections along with food and changing the site of injection frequently.

General Guidelines on Insulin Use

Insulin is mainstay of treatment in approximately 1/3rd of patients of diabetes. However, unless the patient is equipped with the knowledge and know how, the desired results cannot be obtained. Hence, the patient's education in various aspects of diabetes and its control is vital.

Storage

Insulin is ideally stored in a refrigerator at 2°-8°C. Insulin should not be kept in the freezer or exposed to extremes of temperature. The commercially available insulin can be kept at room temperatures for 6 to 8 weeks. Insulin vials after expiry date should never be used.

Strength

Insulin are available in 40 IU/ml or 100 IU/ml strengths. It is essential to use the appropriate syringe for them.

Insulin Injection Technique

It is advisable to gently shake the suspension before use. The vial can be rolled gently upside down and sideways between the hands to ensure uniform suspension. Then vial is turned upside down and air is injected by syringe. The amount of air injected should be equivalent to the units of insulin to be withdrawn.

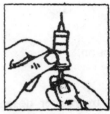

Draw air into the syringe in an amount corresponding to the prescribed dose of cloudy insulin.

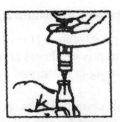

Inject the air into the vial containing the cloudy insulin—but do not draw up insulin!

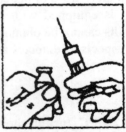

Pull out the needle and put the vial aside.

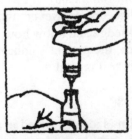

Draw air into the syringe in an amount corresponding to the prescribed dose of clear insulin and inject the air into the vial containing clear insulin.

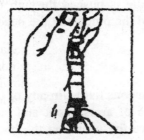

Invert the vial and draw up clear insulin—a little more than prescribed.

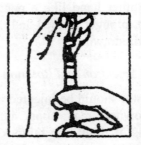

Hold the vial vertically at eye level Inject the excess amount of insulin, together with any air bubbles, back into the vial. Pull out the needle

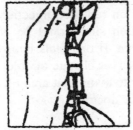

Now take the vial containing cloudy insulin and air. Insert the needle and draw up the accurate amount of insulin prescribed.

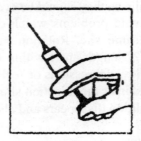

Pull out the needle. Now, the mixture is ready for use.

The Insulin vials which require mixing are usually of Plain/ Regular (clear vial) and Lente/NPH (cloudy vial). For mixing insulins first clean the rubber stopper of each bottle with spirit swab, then with the syringe, draw the air equivalent to level of desired units of Lente (cloudy) Insulin, later repeat the same for dose of Plain/Regular Insulin (clear). Ensure that there is not bubble in the syringe, (if present gently tap the syringe, to push the bubble to the top and then force it in the bottle).

Injection Technique

Clean the site selected with the spirit swab, then skin is gently pinched between the thumb and forefinger, hold the syringe with the other hand like a pencil and needle is pushed through the skin, plunger pushed and then released the pinch and the needle is withdrawn.

Site Selection and Rotation

Insulin should be injected into subcutaneous tissue, in any of the following areas: upper and outer area of arms, front and side areas of thigh, the buttocks, just above the waist, on the back, abdomen except the areas around the umblicus and at the waistline. The accidental intramuscular injection is painful and can cause tissue scaring. Factors like massage, increases exercise of the area where insulin injection is given can alter the absorption of insulin so they should be avoided. Rotation of the side is important to avoid problems which could occur on repeated injections at the same site. Rotation of the injection site should be about 1-1/2" length apart within the same area. If one feels lumps, or shallow depressions or feel pain or observes change of colour of the skin at the injection site, it is better to avoid that area till that condition disappears and also consult the doctor.

Timing

Insulin should be injected 30 to 45 minutes before the meals so that its onset of action corresponds to the rise in Blood Sugar that occurs with the meals.

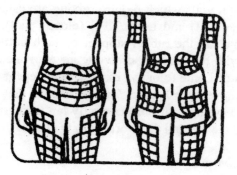

Site Selection and Rotation

Insulin and Exercise

Exercise can be associated with hypoglycemia in patients on insulin. Patient should make necessary adjustments in their meal plans or insulin regimen on the days of exercise in consultation with their doctor.

Insulin and Illness

Illness can disrupt diabetic control. However, the problems can be minimised. If the patients follows basic guidelines:

1. Do not stop the insulin injection,
2. Continue testing the Blood Sugar, urine sugar, for ketones,
3. Adapt your eating patterns to more easily tolerated foods, and
4. Food should be taken as frequently in short intervals.

If the above simple precautions are observed by the patients who use insulin, many of their day to day problems can be avoided.

Pancrease Transplantation

Here pancrease gland of other person is transplanted into Diabetic patients. There are many problems like availability of donor and rejection of graft by body.

Insulin Pumps

An insulin pump is a battery-powered, computerized device about the size of a deck of cards. Inside the pump is a syringe of short-acting insulin with a gear-driven plunger. A thin tube, 21 to 43 inches long, is attached to the pump. At the other end of the tube is a needle or catheter. You insert the needle or catheter under your skin, usually in your abdomen or thigh. Insulin is delivered through the tube and needle or catheter into your body.

You programme the pump. You tell it how much insulin you want and when you want it. You tell the pump to give you tiny amounts of short-acting insulin continuously throughout the day and night, just the way a normal pancrease would. Then you tell the pump to give you extra insulin just before you eat.

Your wear an insulin pump pretty much all the time, either inside or outside your clothes. A pump may be water-proof or come with a water-proof case for showers and swimming.

You can, of course, take the pump off. If you'll have the pump off for more than 1 hour, you may need a short of short-acting insulin. Check your blood glucose to be sure. Yes, you still need to test your blood glucose. At least four tests a day are recommended.

What the Pump can do for You

Get your blood glucose level closer to normal. This is called tight control. If your insulin shots have not controlled your blood glucose levels, in insulin pump might work better for you.

Smooth out blood glucose swings. If you have frequent blood glucose swings, the insulin pump can help smooth them out.

Take care of the night-time lows and the morning highs. Your body need less insulin at night than at dawn. If you try to lower the dose of your evening insulin shot to avoid low blood glucose at night, you won't enough insulin in the morning. Then you'll have high blood glucose when you wake up.

With an insulin pump, you can programme it to give you less insulin at night and more insulin before dawn. That way you avoid night-time low blood glucose and morning high blood glucose.

Be Aware

Ketoacidosis. When your body has too little or no insulin, you risk getting ketoacidosis. Ketoacidosis is a dangerous buildup of ketones in your blood.

If the tube to your insulin pumps gets blocked or twisted or the needle comes out, you won't be getting insulin, and you may not know it. (Pumps do have alarms that signal when the tube is blocked, the insulin is low, or the battery is low. But they don't signal when the needle has come out.)

Ketones can start to build up in 1 hour. Ketoacidosis can develop in as little as 6 hours. Your best protection is to check your blood glucose levels often. If your blood glucose level is over 250mg/dl, check your urine for ketones.

Infection. The place where the needle or catheter enters your body may become infected. To lessen your chances of infection, clean the area before your insert the needle or catheter, change sites within the area every 48 hours (See Insulin Shots), and use an antibiotic ointment and protective cover.

Skin allergy. You may have an allergic reaction around the needle or catheter site. Try non-allergenic tape or Teflon catheters.

Costs and Insurance

Pumps cost between $3,000 and $5,000. Supplies for a month, including blood glucose monitoring strips, cost about $300.

If you think you may want a pump, talk to your doctor. Learning how to use a pump can take some time. Your doctor may want you to be in the hospital for a few days when you first get a pump so that you can learn all about how to use it.

In India it is not available at present but few people who got it from abroad are using. By next year it would be available but the cost factor and maintenance would be a problem.

Spontaneous Hypoglycaemia

Some people have a tendency to develop low blood sugar levels which can cause extreme weakness. In a normal person, fasting blood sugar levels are 70 to 100mg/100ml and 2 hours after food, blood sugar levels are between 100 to 140mg/100ml.

Some of these persons get up in the morning with headache and weakness which gets better with tea. Two hours after breakfast, they again get the feeling of *Ghabrahat*, palpitation, sweating and restlessness (Funny Turns) and these symptoms persist till the person eats something. These symptoms are due to low blood glucose—medical name is hypoglycemia. Blood sugar level are usually less than 60mg/100ml.

Many people may be suffering from this condition but they are rarely diagnosed. Most of the time these patients are diagnosed having heart problems and referred to cardiologist or referred to psychiatrist for the treatment of depressions or anxiety.

If the blood sugar is tested during these episodes, it would be below the normal range, i.e. usually less then 60mg/100ml.

Large number of otherwise normal people occasionally become pale, weak, sweaty (sweating) when meals are due and such people report benefit from advice to take regular snacks between meals. True hypoglycemia may develop after food in the presence of alcohol which stimulates 'B' cells of pancreas gland to produce exaggerated response to carbohydrates. Persons who consume alchoholic beverages like Beer or other alcoholic drink in place of lunch are potentially at risk of developing hypoglycaemia.

The feelings people have when they are having low blood sugar are due to two things. First, the Brain itself cannot work properly when the blood glucose fall below 55 mg/100 ml and secondly, the body reacts to low blood glucose by producing hormones (mainly adrenalin) which increases blood glucose.

When Brain is affected, it causes

* Weakness of legs
* Double/blurred vision
* Confusion
* Headache
* Drowsiness

Adrenalin hormone—causes

* Sweating
* Rapid heart beat
* Feeling of panic and anxiety

Most people find it hard to describe how they feel but the proof is that the blood glucose is low.

What can cause hypoglycaemia

Common cause

* People who take medicines for control of Diabetes
* People who take anti-malarials or pain killers frequently
* Alcohol can cause hypoglycaemia specially in the early morning if food was not taken along with drinks in the night.

How to Prevent

Most important aspect is correction of diet. Modification of eating habits may help in resolving this problem. Change in lifestyle and behavioural modification may also help in correcting it.

One should avoid concentrated sugars/carbohydrates because 2 hours after consuming these preparations there is again rebound hypoglycaemia. By using concentrated carbohydrate preparations there is over production of insulin which further reduces blood sugar levels.

What to do

1. Avoid refined sugar, i.e. Sugar, Jaggery, Honey, Jam,

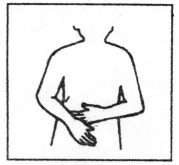

Hunger Pains

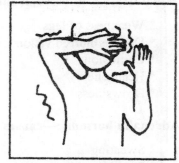

Trembling and Sweating

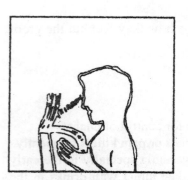

Blurred Vision

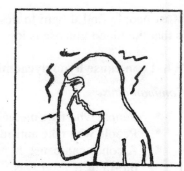

Headache

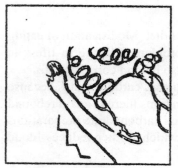

Giddiness

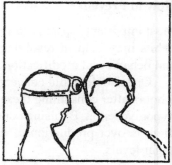

If you have all these Symptoms
Contact Doctor

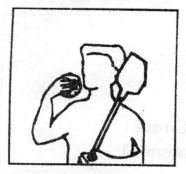

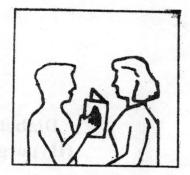

Eat something before Exercise   Keep Family Members
informed about Symptoms of
Hypoglycaemia

chocolates, Sweet Potatoes and Biscuits.

2. Can use complex carbohydrates which include fruits, cereals and vegetables like papaya, cereals, pulses, pumpkin etc.

3. Food with high fibre content can be used. Beans and peas may be consumed frequently.

4. Frequent small meals may help in keeping blood sugar levels in normal range. Regular exercise especially aerobic ones will help in preventing extra weight gain.

5. Alcohol should be avoided. If one can't resist this, he should not take more than one or two drinks (30 ml each), that too over a period of 3 to 4 hours time along with snacks followed by meals/dessert.

6. Smoking during these episodes should be avoided as it may increase the problem by increasing heart beat, sweating and trembling.

7. Avoid sweets, ice cream and chocolates as they will increase weight.

8. Most persons take sugar, glucose, sweets to get rid of this problem but it rebounces/relapses because there is great insulin release which produces hypoglycaemia. So one should avoid sugar mixers. Persons having symptoms of low blood sugar should avoid religious fastings.

Diabetic Coma
(Hyperglycaemia)

Diabetic Coma, Ketoacidosis

When Blood Sugar levels are high patient becomes dull, extreme weakness, vomiting feels sleepy, skin is dry and breathlessness Drowsy and unconscious and coma.

Warning signs

— If one gets more and more desire for food and thirst.
— Increased frequency of micturition.
— Sudden Loss of Weight.
— Feeling more sleepy and drowsy than usual.
— Vomiting and pain in Abdomen.
— Smell of over riped fruits in breath.
— Fast and deep breathing. If Blood Sugar is above 400mg%.
— Urine examination will reveal ketones.

Why this Happens (Seen under following circumstances)

1. If diabetic patients eat more and more and irregular in taking medicines.
2. Usually seen in Type I Diabetes, in children who may forget to take Insulin or during some infections when Blood Sugar levels will rise very rapidly.
3. It can be seen in Adults too during stressful situations, infections or in persons who are alcoholic and absolutely irregular in taking medicines and food.

Symptoms

1. Excessive thirst.
2. Appetite.
3. Urination and weakness.
4. Dry skin.
5. Breathlessness.
6. Pain in Abdomen and distension.
7. Vomiting.
8. Nausea.
9. Drowsiness.
10. Disorientation and unconsciousness and coma. Blood Sugar Test will reveal very high Blood sugar.

Urine will show—ketones (Normal urine will not show ketones)

Prevention and Treatment

All diabetic patients should know about hyperglycaemia and diabetic coma. Parents and relatives should be told about warning signs of diabetic coma. So that appropriate steps could be taken to prevent it. Patients should be shifted to hospital immediately where proper treatment can be given.

Insulin therapy along with other measures can save the life. So delay in shifting patient to good Medical Centre/Hospital should be avoided.

Hyperglycaemia (High Blood Sugar)

Causes

1. Not enough medication.
2. Too much carbohydrate.
3. Increase in weight.
4. Lack of activity.
5. Illness.
6. Stress.
7. Excessive urination.
8. Excessive thirst.

9. Tiredness.
10. Blurred vision.
11. Recurrent infections and slow healing.

Management

1. Check medications or seek medical advice.
2. Review diet.
3. Review diet and activity level.
4. Seek medical advice.
5. Review causes of stress.

❏   Diabectic ketoacidosis is an emergency.
❏   Do not take it lightly. Contact your doctor immediately.
    Symptoms are:
    ● Excessive, urination and thirst
    ● Nausea, vomiting and abdominal pain
    ● Deep, rapid breathing with a fruity smell
    ● Mental confusion.
❏   Blood/urine testing will reveal high sugar levels and presence of ketones.

Diabetes Ketoacidosis in Children

* If your diabetes is untreated or poorly controlled, blood glucose levels rise very high (hyperglycaemia).
* This occurs because you don't have enough insulin for your needs, the glucose in the blood is not being taken into the cells so your body makes its own fuel by burning up stored fat.
* When fat is used in this way, waste products called ketones are produced and these excreted in the urine.
* Small amounts of ketones are not harmful, and are normally produced when you start to burn up body fat...for example when you go on a weight reduction diet.

However, problems arise when Blood Sugar levels are high and excessive ketones are produced and these start to accumulate in the body.

If untreated this will result in a condition called 'ketoacidosis'.

This condition is serious and urgent medical treatment is essential.

What causes this?

1. Illness and infection (e.g. flu, vomiting, diarrhoea, urine infections).
2. Missed or incorrect insulin dosage.
3. Poor injection technique.
4. Ineffective insulin due to faulty storage or expired date.

Watch for

1. The common signs and symptoms of hyperglycaemia, e.g. excessive urination and thirst, dry mouth and skin, tiredness.

2. Persistant high level of sugar in blood or urine.
3. Presence of ketones in the urine.
4. Nausea, vomiting and abdominal pain.
5. Sweet smell of acetone in the breath.
6. Respiration—deep and rapid.
7. Altered levels of consciousness.

To Prevent Ketoacidosis

If your are sick

1. Take your usual dose of insulin.
2. Test your Blood Sugar level and urine ketones at least 4 hourly (or more often if necessary).
3. Contact your Doctor with your results.
4. Give extra quick acting insulin according to your doctor's guidelines.

   If you cannot contact your Doctor, follow these guidelines:

   (a) If your Blood Sugar Level (BSL) is less than 260 mg/100ml, continue your normal insulin.

   (b) If your Blood Sugar Level (BSL) is between 260 mg% to 360 mg% give 4 units of quick acting insulin (Hum insulin-r or Actrapid) every 4 hours, in addition to your usual dose.

   (c) If your Blood Sugar Level (BSL) is above 360 mg/100 ml, give 4 units of quick acting insulin (Hum Insulin-r or Actrapid) every 2 hours, in addition to your usual dose.

   (d) Follow this procedure until your BSL is less than 250mg/100ml of Blood.

5. If you don't feel like eating, replace your normal carbohydrate portions with simple carbohydrate fluids, fruit juice etc. if your Blood Sugar Level (BSL) is persistently above 250mg/100ml, sip unsweetened fluids only.

6. Take extra clear sugar-free fluids. You need to have 200-500ml/hour (depending on your body size and degree of dehydration).
7. If your BSL is persistently high or if you are vomiting, you must contact your Doctor or go to Hospital.

Do not Delay!

Children with diabetes are no more likely to develop sore throats or virus illnesses than any other child providing their diabetes is well controlled. When diabetes is first diagnosed, poorly controlled, during an infection, stress, or other illness, the body's need for insulin increases. This causes the Blood Sugar level to rise very high (hyperglycaemia). With this lack of insulin the body cells can no longer use the glucose as the main source of energy so the body makes its own fuel by burning up stored fats. When fat is used in this way, waste products called ketones are produced and these are excreted in the urine.

High Blood Sugar	+	Reduced Insulin	=	Stored Fat	→ Ketones
	Pancreas				→ Energy

However, a problem arises when Blood Sugar levels are high and excessive ketones are produced and these start to accumulate in the body. If untreated this will result in.

Ketoacidosis

This condition is serious and urgent medical treatment is essential.

Causes

1. Initial diagnosis.
2. Illness and infection (e.g. flu, vomiting, diarrhoea).
3. Missed or incorrect insulin dosage (including poor injection technique).
4. Long-term poor control and neglect.

Watch For

1. The common signs and symptoms of hyperglycaemia.
    — Excessive urination;
    — Thirst;
    — Tiredness;
    — Weight loss;
    — Signs of dehydration
      • dry mouth/skin;
      • sunken eyes.
2. Persistent high levels of Sugar in the blood or urine.
3. Presence of ketones in the urine.
4. Nausea, vomiting and abdominal pains, vomiting is always serious.
5. Sweet small of acetone on the breath.
6. Respirations and rapid.
7. Altered level of consciousness.

These symptoms may develop over hours or days.

PREVENTING KETOACIDOSIS IN CHILDREN

To Prevent ketoacidosis

If you are sick

1. *Never Omit Insulin*—always take your usual dose.
2. *Test Blood Sugar and Urine Ketones*—Atleast every 2 hours and hourly is necessary.
3. *Contact Your Doctor*—give results of tests.
4. *Extra Insulin*—quick acting insulin may be needed according to your doctor's guidelines.

If you cannot contact your doctor follow these guidelines:

(a) If your Blood Sugar Level (BSL) is less than 200mg%, continue your normal insulin;

(b) If your BSL is between 280-360mg per 100 ml of

Blood, give 2 units of quick acting insulin (Hum Insulin-r or Actrapid) every 4 hours, in addition to your usual dose;

(c) If your BSL is above 360mg/100ml of Blood, give 2 units of quick acting insulin every 2 hours in addition to your usual dose;

(d) Follow this procedure until your BSL is less than 280 mg%.

5. *Replace Normal Carbohydrate*—If you don't feel like eating, replace with simple carbohydrate fluids, e.g. flat ordinary lemonade, fruit juice etc. (see your sick day card). If your BSL is persistently above 15mmol/L sip carbohydrate free (unsweetened) fluids (lemon juice mineral water).

6. *Extra Fluids*—You need to have extra carbohydrate free fluids every hour. (The amount depends on body size and degree of dehydration.)

7. *High BSL or Vomiting*—If BSL persistently high or you are vomiting you must contact your doctor or go to hospital.

Obesity or Over Weight

What is Obesity?

Obesity is the excessive accumulation of body fat, i.e. more than 25% of ideal body weight in boys and 32% in girls. Worldwide, 51% of women, 44% of men and 30% of children are overweight. At least one child in five is obese.

How do you come to know Whether you are Overweight, Obese or Normal Weight?

There is a scale called Body Mass Index (BMI) Which is calculated from height and weight. This differs in male and female and for different age groups. The charts for the calculation can be availed.

Why do you become obese or overweight?

* Genetic — Family history of obesity or overweight
* Environmental

- Sedentary lifestyle (No/minimal physical activity in daily life, watching TV, playing video games, working on computers, etc.)

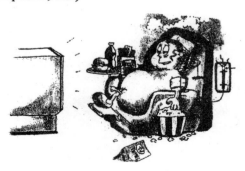

- Food Habits (Eating high fat, low fiber and high quantity (calories) diet like Burgers, Pizzas, French fries, Cola drinks, etc.).

What can you do about it?

If you are not obese, not over weight.....Prevent both!
If you are over weight.......Reduce your weight and prevent obesity!
If your are obese.....Get ride or it!

How to get rid of Obesity?

Can be changed   *Can't be changed*
* Food Habits   * Genetic Background
* Physical activities

Obesity Leads—Diabetes in children, Hypertension in children, Joints problems in children.

Step by Step....

Food Habits —   Eat the quantity (calories) only as much is needed for your daily activity. Neither less nor more.
Choose food high in fiber, low in fat which will help in controlling the quantity too.

Physical activity — Do physical activity which will consume calories on a regular basis. Use the leisure times for out door games instead of being Couch Potato.

Role of Teachers/School

- Planned, systematic inculcation of the above habits into children. Allocating certain fixed hours for guidance on nutrition in the curriculum.
- Discouraging the fast food outlets inside the school

premises.
- Distribution of healthy dietary information for parents through children.
- Organizing dietary seminars for parents in the school.
- Encouraging healthy dietary stalls in school meals and annual functions.
- Encouraging children and giving awards to those children, who participate in Physical activity and Games.

Role of Parents

Children see their parents as their "Role Models" in life, hence it is of utmost importance to:

- Set examples by making healthy food choices and practicing physical activities at home on an ongoing basis.
- Explain the values of each food items and activities to children as much as possible.

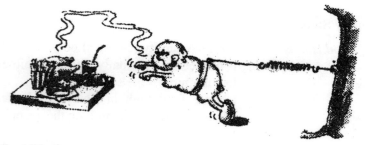

Most Strange

It does seem strange however that there are campaigns against smoking, drinking and yet obesity which poses as a serious threat to life is brushed under the Carpet. It is not a "Sociable Topic".

That's why we thought of this project "Obesity Prevention At Grassroots Level."

"Never sit it you can stand
Never Stand it You can Walk
Never Walk if you can Run"

Diabetes and Heart Problems

One of the commonest causes of heart attack is diabetes mellitus and in majority of diabetes patients cause of death is heart attack. There are certain peculiarities of heart attack in these patients, as compare to heart attacks in non-diabetic patients.

— Incidence of heart attack in diabetics is higher than general public.

— Incidence of heart attacks in diabetic males is 50 times higher while in females it is 10 times more.

— Incidence of sudden death due to Sudden Cardiac Arrest is 50 times more in males, while it is 300 times more in females in diabetics.

— 35% of diabetic patients die due to heart problems before they reach the 55 years of age as compare to 4 to 8% of general public.

— 50% Diabetic patients have high blood pressure.

In obese diabetic patients blood cholesterol and triglyceride levels are high and these get deposited in the blood vessels which supply blood to heart. Because of this deposition blood supply is affected (due to narrowing of blood vessels) and this can cause Angina or Heart Attack.

Other additional factors are:

— Obesity—Over weight.

— High Blood Pressure.

— Smoking.

— Blood vessels of legs, foot and arms also get narrowed down due to cholesterol deposition and can cause pain in legs while walking which may become better by further walking. This is seen more frequently in Diabetics who are smoker.

Precautions

Certain precautions are essential—

— Weight Records—reduce over weight.
— Control Blood Pressure.
— Swelling over legs and feet should be reported to Doctor.
— Get regular sugar and cholesterol examinations and keep records.
— Get X-Ray chest once in a year.
— Get E.C.G. once in a year.
— If one gets discomfort in chest while walking or after food should undergo stress test/tread mill test so that cadiac status can be evaluated.

Bad Companions of Diabetes

• Hypertension (High Blood Pressure)
• Dyslipidaemia (High Cholesterol and Triglyceride Levels)
• Smoking
• Obesity (Over Weight) *Motapa*

All the above factors increase the risk for Strokes and Heart Attacks.

Hypertension (High Blood Pressure) is associated with:

— Insulin Resistance,
— Obesity Central, and
— Accelerated Atherosclerosis (Blockage of artry).

By keeping Blood Pressure under control there was large reduction of stroke, i.e. by 44%.

Blood Pressure should be kept around 130/82 to prevent vascular complication of Diabetes mainly stroke and heart attacks.

As 40% of diabetics have associated with high blood pressure, all diabetic patients should have regular blood pressure check up and if needed use medicines regularly as per their doctors advice.

Diabetic Heart Attack are seen in young diabetic and are usually severe. Heart Attack are painless (silent). Usually seen in the age group of 35 to 40 years. All the major blood vessels of Heart are involved. Always need By-Pass Surgery.

Instead of pain they get discomfort in chest, suffocation and difficulty in breathing.

How to Cope
— Stop smoking.
— Keep Blood Sugar under control.
— Regular exercise and weight control.
— Control Blood Pressure.
— Regular Heart check up an follow your Doctor's advise.

By-Pass Surgery
— Diabetes involves heart muscle and Blood vessels of heart and reduces expectancy of life.
— By-Pass Surgery would improve the quality of life make change in food habits and lifestyle.
— Persons can lead normal life.

Diabetes and Pregnancy

Diabetes does not spare anyone, let it be young or old, male or female, pregnant or non-pregnant female. Many years ago if a female was having many abortions, or was delivering abnormal or dead child it was presumed as God's *will*.

After many years of research and investigations the actual cause was identified. It is uncontrolled diabetes during pregnancy which is one of the causes of abortions.

Normally pregnant ladies have low levels of fasting blood sugar as compare to post prandial blood sugar which are little higher than normal.

Usually in pregnancy Insulin secretion is more but due to deficiency or defective production of Insulin diabetes develops in pregnancy.

Growth of the organs of child usually takes place in 1st three months of pregnancy. I during this period Blood Sugar remains high child will have congenital defects, like valvular heart defects absence of some parts of body or organs.

In other words pregnancy should be planned only once you are sure that there is no diabetes.

Uncontrolled diabetes in 2nd and 3rd trimester of pregnancy can cause mental retardation of child, size of head would be bigger and overall size of child may be big. Then mother can't deliver such child normally and she has to go under Caesarian operation.

Therefore to avoid all this urine and blood tested for sugar.

Which group of ladies should undergo screening for Blood Sugar.

— All females with family history of diabetes.
— If urine sample shows sugar.
— H/o repeated abortions or still birth.
— H/o delivery of abnormal size children.
— H/o delivery of child with congenital deformity.

Special blood test is available to detect the Blood Sugar Level pattern of last 2-3 months. This is done by estimation of Glycosylated haemoglobin. This test is specially helpful in planning motherhood and would indicate about the Blood Sugar Levels at the time of conception and before that.

Gestational Diabetes

What is gestational diabetes?

— Diabetes occurring for the first time in pregnancy.
— Onset is usually mid to late pregnancy.
— More common in those women:
  • whose relatives have diabetes
  • who are over 30 years
  • who are over weight

Why is it so important to maintain strict control of Blood Sugar?

— Poor diabetes control is associated with the risk of large babies with difficult labour.
— These babies may then have breathing problems and low Blood Sugar Levels at birth.
— Good diabetes control means a normal pregnancy and a normal delivery, with a healthy baby.

How will I know if my baby is doing well?

— Your Obstetrician will closely monitor your baby's progress. The baby's growth and development will be measured by Ultrasound.
— With good diabetes control you can expect a *normal* labour and delivery. Sometimes, it is necessary to induce labour a little earlier. If the baby is too big a Caesarian Section may be necessary.
— After the birth, your baby will be watched closely in the Special Care Nursery for 24 to 48 hours to ensure the Blood Sugar Levels stay normal.

— Your baby will not be born with diabetes.

Should I take any special precautions after my pregnancy?

— You should have a Glucose Tolerance Test after the birth of your baby, to ensure a return to normal has once a year.
— Have a Blood Sugar Level done at least once a year.
— Be aware that you have a greater risk of developing Gestational Diabetes in future pregnancies.
— You have a greater risk developing Diabetes later in life (usually non-insulin dependent diabetes).

Is there anything I can do to prevent diabetes in later life?

— Continue with your diet (after adjustment by a Dietitian).
— Maintain ideal body weight for your height.
— Exercise to stay fit.

How to Manage

One should plan delivery only in hospital in such cases so that life of both mother and child can be saved.

Ultrasound examination will help to find out if there is any congenital defect so that appropriate precaution may be taken.

In Type II diabetes pregnant lady is aware about her being diabetic still she is reluctant to stop tablets. Pregnant ladies should not take any tablets for diabetes because these tablets are harmful to (Foetus) child. Only safe and best treatment available is regular injection of Insulin. Pregnant diabetic lady requires one or two injections of plane Insulin. Newer available humane insulins are safe. Patient may require one or two injections depending upon Blood Sugar Levels.

Other factors are also essential in the treatment apart from insulin injections.

About Diet

In pregnant lady there is increase in weight per week, in the

range of 300-400gm.
- Food should provide proper nutrition to both mother and child for growth.
- Should not increase extra weight.
- Should keep Blood Sugar Levels under control.
- Should provide 30-40 calories per kg. of normal weight.

Exercise—Should go for regular walk.

Diabetes and Eyes

One of the most important and sensitive organ of the body is Eyes. In diabetes eyes like any other organ of body are involved and can cause complete blindness.

Involvement of eyes depend upon the duration of diabetes. If diabetes is there for more than 15 years eyes are definitely involved.

Eyes are more involved in Type I diabetes than Type II diabetes. Other factor which is responsible for eye involvement is uncontrolled Blood Sugar. Prolonged period of uncontrolled diabetes causes more danger to eyes.

Symptoms are

— Itching in eyes, irritation.
— Watering, painful eye movements.
— Headache, redness, diminished vision.
— Double vision, black spots in front of eyes.
— Frequent change in power of glasses.
— Paralysis of eye muscles leading to double vision or squint.
— Cataract, and sudden loss of vision—due to bleeding in eye or retinal detachment.

How to Manage

Best and simple way to keep the diabetes under control is by strict diet control and regular use of anti-diabetic medicines.

— All diabetic patients should have regular complete eye check up at least once in a year.
— Diabetics who smoke are at a higher risk for loss of eye sight.
— Blood pressure should be kept under control.
— Retinal detachment and retinopathy can be kept under

control by photo coagulation and laser therapy which is very effective. This type of treatment is available at all big centres. It is prophylactic therapy and can prevent blindness in Diabetic patients.

Eye Care in Diabetes

When you have diabetes, you have a high risk of eye problems that can lead to severe damage or blindness. This risk becomes even higher if you are between 40 to 60 years old age if you have had diabetes for a number of years.

What is especially bad is that many times the eyes are damaged before any symptoms are felt. So it is very important to visit your eye doctor regularly (at least once a year)—and immediately if you notice anything wrong with your eyes.

Common Diabetics Eye Problems

1. *Cataracts*—Clouding of the normally clear lens in the eye.
2. *Glaucoma*—An increase in pressure within the eye.
3. *Diabetic retinopathy*—Weakening and breaking down of the small blood vessels in the retain.

Eye Care Do's	*Eye Care Don'ts*
• Wear goggles or safety glasses if eyes are at risk.	• Don't touch eyes with dirty fingers.
• Direct all spray nozzles away from eyes.	• Don't rub or overuse eyes.
• Read instructions on liquids or Powders.	• Don't sit under sun-lamp without goggles.
• Wear sun glasses on bright days (especially on sand, or snow).	• Don't use saliva to wet makeup or contact lenses.
• Get immediate treatment for red/painful eyes.	• Don't wear dirty contact lenses.
• Tell eye specialists you have diabetes.	• Don't try to remove particles from eyes; see a physician.

Dental Care in Diabetes

The most common major oral complication of diabetes is gum (periodontal) disease. In untreated, Diabetes gum disease can be very serious and lead to tooth loss.

Early warning signs of gum disease include : long-term bad breath or bad taste; swollen, red, tender, shrinking, or bleeding gums; pus between teeth; changes in bite, teeth position, or denture fit; and tooth loss.

* Brush and floss after every meal and before bed time.
* Use of soft-bristled brush and unwaxed floss.
* Brush all surfaces of all teeth.
* Lightly brush your tongue.
* Massage your gums gently with finger or brush.
* Use fluoride tooth-paste.
* Eat a well-balanced diet.
* Avoid foods high in sugar, especially foods that stick to teeth like raisins, caramel, and other chewy candies.
* Visit your Dentist every three months for cleaning, polishing, inspection, and oral hygiene instruction.

Nerve Involvement in Diabetes

Diabetes involves all the nerves and muscles of body. Numbness in feet, tingling, burning, sensations, pain in legs specially at night are all features of diabetic Neuropathy. Some patients will not be able to walk due to pain in legs or weakness once they sit down they can't get up without support.

Some people may feel difficulty in typing or writing and all movements of body become painful.

These are all signs of involvement of Nerves called as Neuropathy or Diabetic Neuritis. This damage is due to poor control and longer durations of diabetes. These symptoms are both Sensory (Burning, tingling, numbness) and Motor (weakness and wasting of muscles).

All these symptoms, i.e. Sensory and Motor are the result of uncontrolled Diabetes and patient usually responds well once Blood Sugar is controlled either by Medicines or by Insulin injections.

Some persons may have diminished sweating in the feet or increased sweating over upper part of body.

Some persons will have constipation. Others will have intermittent watery diarrhoea especially at night or other will have distension of abdomen.

Some Diabetic patients have Urinary and sexual problems also like:

— Difficulty in passing urine.
— Repeated urine infections.
— Difficulty in holding urine.

Impotence, i.e. unability to achieve or sustain erection satisfactorily for sexual intercourse. This is one of the commonest problem, diabetic patient face. Yet for months and years they won't discuss it with their doctor. Most of the time either doctor is too busy or patient is with family members so he is not able to express the problem to doctor. Longer the duration of uncontrolled Diabetes more and more would be Sexual problems. Some patients may request their doctor for some magic pill or injection. Some people may try Alcohol or other drugs—but all these may aggravate the agony of patient.

Treatment

1. Psychological counselling to both partners.
2. Stop use of Alcohol.
3. Strict Diabetes control.
4. There are certain devices—suction technique erection can be maintained—(suction pumps are available).
5. Injections of Papaverine before intercourse can cause sustained erection. However, these all techniques have side effects of infections etc., and should be under strict medical supervision.

For all Neruological problems arising due to uncontrolled diabetes the best treatment is to keep Blood Sugar under control and consult your doctor before trying for any magic pill.

Skin and Sexual Problems in Diabetes

Skin Problems

About 30 to 35% of Diabetic patients develop skin problems. Because of Diabetes the severity of these infections is more as compare to the Non-Diabetic.

Diabetic patients develop finger infections of Nails, Nail bed, between fingers, inner and part of thigh or at private parts. Some time itching and rash may be presenting symptom of Diabetes in females specially if she is over weight. In males cuts at glans penis indicate increase in Blood Sugar.

Sometimes Diabetic patient will have oral ulcers or thrush. Fingers infection of Nails may cause swelling and performation at one side of Nail or destruction of Nail. Sometimes there are ulcers between fingers or toes and it may be so much painful that one cannot wear shoes.

Diabetic men present with redness and swelling of the penis at opening and it is usually associated with sever itching and pain. This is called as Balanitis. There may be difficulty in retracting skin.

In some Diabetic patients because of these problems circumcision is advised.

In all above skin problems antifungal lotions and creams help in solving the problem. All above conditions indicate that the Blood Sugar is not under control and it has to be kept in control.

Sexual Problems in Diabetes

Diabetes is one of the few diseases that can cause impotence, i.e. loss of the ability to achieve and maintain an erection hard enough for sexual intercourse—also called as Erectile Dysfunction (ED).

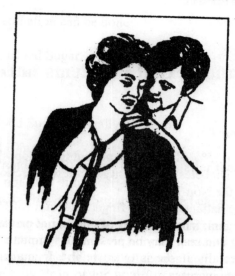

Erectile Dysfunction is 3 times more common among diabetics than in the healthy control population. Incidence varies from 28 to 59%.

Predictive Factors

Age, duration of diabetes, levels of Blood Sugar presence of complications especially Retinopathy and Neuropathy, high blood pressure and drugs taken for controlling it, smoking and alcohol abuse. Risk of impotence is high in diabetics where Blood Sugar are on very high side and HbA_{IC} is more than 9.8%. Persistent high blood glucose leads to certain chemical changes which damage arteries and nerves.

Initially, there is diminished Penile rigidity and reduced ability to sustain an erection. This progress to full-fledged failure of Erection. Very often, sexual desire persists.

Psychological factors

There is substantial evidence to suggest that Erectile Dysfunction in diabetes is often Psychological in origin. Factors are: awareness

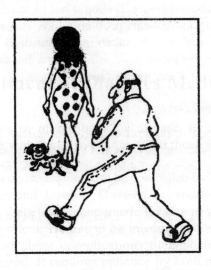

of suffering from a chronic condition, relationship problems and fear of failure during sexual intercourse. Many patients don't discuss this problem with their doctor. Only 50% of diabetics having sexual problems discuss with their doctor about it.

How to Manage

First and the most important aspect of treatment is to control Blood Sugar by diet or drug treatment and by persuading the patient to abstain from risk factors like smoking and alcohol abuse.

Psychotherapy care help to minimize the anxiety and modify the couple's sexual habits in helpful way.

Drug treatment

Many drugs are being used for correcting this disorder. SILDENAFIL (VIAGRA now available in Indian Market also) is very effective in controlling Erctile Dysfunctions in diabetic men. It relaxes smooth muscles, increases blood flow and this leads to penile erection.

Medicine is taken 60 minute before intercourse and has an

effect lasting about 4 hours. It should not be taken by men taking Nitrates for angina or heart problems like, isosorbide, dinitrate, monotrate etc. It should be taken only after discussion with your doctor. Other common side effects are headache, flushing, stomache and meld temporary visual changes.

Other Drugs and Devices

Certain hormonal treatment or anti-depressants are also useful. Self injection, vacuum devices and surgical implants are the other therapeutics options available which your doctor would suggest to you.

FREQUENTLY ASKED QUESTIONS FOR ERECTILE DYSFUNCTION (ED)

Sexual Problems in Diabetes by Men

Q. 1. What is an Erectile Dysfunction?

Ans. Erectile Dysfunction is the persistent inability for a man to achieve and maintain an erection for a complete and satisfactory sexual activity. Previously it was also called as impotence, which had negative connotation. But, now the term used is Erectile Dysfunction which describes the medical problem more accurately and with a precise clinical description.

Q. 2. How Common is ED among Men?

Ans. Do not panic if you have erectile dysfunction, as you are not the only one suffering. It is a fairly common condition encountered by many. But for a large number of men ED is a frequent problem. An estimated 100 million are affected by this dysfunction.

Q. 3. Does ED Affect the sexual desires?

Ans. No, normally it does not affect the arousal, desire and ejaculation. Erectile Dysfunction means only an inability to obtain or maintain an erection, but has no effect on desire.

Q. 4. Can Erectile Dysfunction be assessed and treated?

Ans. Yes, ED is easily assessed and treated. A detailed history taken from the patient is the most important aspect of diagnosing the ED. For most patients investigation/assessment is limited to bare minimum that is blood pressure and examination of external genitalia. Doctor, will advice you if further tests and investigations are required.

Q.5. What are the treatment options available?

Ans. The treatment option available are intracavernosal prostaglandin injection, transurethral alpostadil, vacuum devices and oral sildenafil therapy. Your physician will advice you on the treatment schedule.

Q.6. Is oral drug therapy effective?

Ans. Oral drug therapy with sildenafil has shown to be effective in treating men with ED. Improvement is erectile response has been observed 50 to 80% if patient.

Q.7. What is sildenafil used for?

Ans. Sildenafil is only used for treatment of men who have difficulty in having and/or maintaining an erection for a complete sexual intercourse, in other words, it is used to treat impotence or erectile dysfunction in men.

Q.8. How does sildenafil action occur in the body?

Ans. An erection is a result of a delicate but perfectly balanced process that involves the brain, blood vessels, nerves and hormones. The penis is specifically designed to respond to the change that occur when a person is sexually aroused. In the penis an erection occurs as a result of an increase in blood flow into the internal area. Sildenafil increases men's ability to achieve and maintain erection during sexual arousal.

Q.9. How to use the medicine?

Ans. The drug sildenafil should be taken an hour before you have sex. It may take longer for the medicine to work if it is taken with a high fat meal. The medicine should be stored at room temperature away from direct light, head and moisture. This medicine should be kept away from children.

Q.10. When the medicine should not be used?

Ans. If you are allergic to sildenafil, than you should not use the drug. It should not be used if you are taking nitrate containing medication that is isosorbide, dinitrate, glyceryl trinitarate etc.

Q. 11. What if I am on some other medication?

Ans. If you are taking some medicine for other ailments, it is best to discuss the problem with your doctor. He will able to advice you.

Q.12. Does sildenafil have any side effects?

Ans. As with most of the drugs some people have side effects others have none. The most common side effect reported by men who have used the drug were: headache, flushing, stomachache and mild and temporary visual changes. If an erection that lasts longer than four hour, which is rare consult your doctor.

Q.13. How many times is the drug taken?

Ans. Sildenafil is used when you want to have an erection. It should be used only one time each day and not more often. Even if you miss a dose it is not harmful as it should be used as and when required or wanted.

Q. 14. Can everyone take Sildenafil?

Ans. Sildenafil is for men who have erectile dysfunction. It will not make a normal erection last longer or occur more often. Therefore, this medicine is not recommended for men who have normal sexual functions.

Q. 15. What about new Drug?

Ans. New drug Tadalafil is now available for use. 10 mg of this salt is taken prior to anticipated sexual activity and without regard to food. Efficacy of Tadalafil persists upto 24 hours post dose.

People with, Angina, Heart Attacks, Low Blood Pressure, Heart Failure and Stroke should not use this Drug.

Diabetes and Kidney Problems

Diabetes and Kidney

Diabetes is one of the most common disease which damages kidney. Every year large number of diabetic patients undergo dialysis and renal transplant. In Type I diabetes 30% patients suffer from Kidney damage if diabetes was detected before the age of 15 years. In NIDDM or Adult type of Diabetes incidence is lower it is about 15 to 20%.

Reasons for involvement of kidney is sustained uncontrolled Blood Sugar. This high Blood Sugar causes changes is Kidney membrane which may lead to excretion of Proteins in urine. Initially very small amount of Albumins (Proteins) is excreted in urine which is called as *Micro-Albuminuria* and which can be detected by special tests. Routine urine test cannot detect such small quantities. Appearance of Albumin in urine indicates early involvement of kidney and usually this stage lasts for many years. It is very important for every Diabetic patient to know about it, because if at this stage Blood Sugar and Blood Pressure are kept under control this process/stage can be reversed. Nature has been so kind with human beings that in this period which should be around 3-5 years if one keeps Blood Sugar under control damage to kidney can be saved.

If Blood Sugar remains high then more and more protein will pass out from urine and symptoms of kidney failure start appearing.

Symptoms

Swelling over eyelids, swelling over feet and legs, nausea, vomiting, *Ghabrahat*, loss of appetite, headache and weakness due to high Blood Pressure, breathlessness, palpitation, and decrease in urine output.

How to Prevent

1. Keep Blood Sugar under control.
2. If Blood Sugar is higher, the damage to kidney will be more so blood pressure should be controlled. Get regular check up and consult your doctor.
3. Proteins restriction is important. If urine start showing albumin reduce protein in take to 20 to 40 gm/day.
4. Don't take medicines without doctor's advice as all medicines have adverse effect on kidneys.
5. Get regular blood test for sugar, urea and creatinine because the results will indicate kidney status.
6. Stop smoking.

Once Renal function shows deterioration then your doctor will advice you for dialysis (Artificial Kidney). Peritoneal or Haemodialysis can help the patient to get rid of toxic products (urea, creatinine) after dialysis. Patient's condition improves. But this cannot be done on permanent basis if repeated dialysis is required then your doctor will advice you to go for Renal transplant.

Renal Transplant

This is successful procedure and routinely performed in our country. It can give a new lease of life to a kidney failure patient and once again patient can lead normal life.

Emergency in Diabetes

There are two types of situations when a Diabetic patient would need urgent medical care.

Hyperglycaemic coma — Very high Blood Sugar levels causing unconsciousness and coma.

Hypoglycaemia — Low Blood Sugar levels—causing unconsciousness and coma.

How a Common Man can Differentiate

Hyperglycaemic coma	*Hypoglycaemic coma*
Excessive thirst	— Excessive Sweating Headache, Palpitation.
Urination, Dry skin Excessive Sugar in Urine	— No sugar in Urine
Urine Test for Ketones (+ve)	— Test for ketones (-ve) (negative).
Extreme weakness and pain in Abdomen	— Trembling.
Rapid and deep breathing	— No change.
Typical smell of over ripe fruits in breath	— Nothing like this.
No response to sugar	— Dissolve sugar and give orally patient becomes normal.
H/O missing injection and excess food intake.	— H/O missing food but taken injection.

Diabetes in Old Age

NIDDM or Type II Diabetes is usually detected in majority of patients between 40 to 70 years of age. As such with advancing age there may be problems of joint pains, impaired vision, impaired hearing, mobility disorders, urinary problems due to enlarged prostate. For a long time he may attribute diabetic symptoms to aging process. It becomes obvious when for some surgery like cataract, or for dental problem he undergoes investigation and then it is revealed that he is suffering from Diabetes. On further questioning he may complain of frequency of urination. He may give a vague history of some family member suffering from Diabetes. As such there are other problems of joint pains, backache, defective vision and uncontrolled diabetes in the presence of these problems become worse.

Due to Diabetes in elderly persons there could be

— lack of Physical strength and impotency.
— Delayed healing of wound and repeated infections.
— High blood pressure, angina or giddiness due to low Blood Pressure.
— Altered Bowel habits constipation or diarrhoea.
— Attacks of pneumonia or urinary infections.

All these problems can be controlled by keeping Blood Sugar under control by proper diet and by regular exercise.

— They should attend Diabetes education camps and should monitor their Diabetes control by getting Blood Sugar or urine sugar examination once or twice weekly.
— Regular exercise 30 to 45 minute walk will not only help in controlling Diabetes but also helps in controlling weight and high blood pressure.

— Diet schedule should be planned. Avoid missing meals or undue exercise which could lead to hypoglycaemia.

— Avoid taking Extra dose of medicine if you have forgotten in the morning as it may cause hypolycaemia (Low Blood Sugar).

— Whenever there is any evidence of cough or chest infection or urinary infection contact your doctor.

— People whose movements are restricted due to arthritis can perform other types of exercises like stretching of arms or limbs to avoid stiffness of joints.

— Constipation or loose motions are the consequences of diabetes so avoid use of strong laxatives. Control of Blood Sugar and use of fiber in diet like ISAFGOL HUSK with water, would help in relieving constipation.

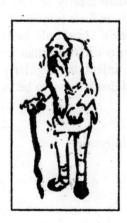

Diabetes in Children

A. Childhood Diabetes

Initially, two to three years, child looks normal but as he grows up he gets more prone to infections. Usually child is hospitalized for some chest or other infections and investigations will reveal that child is having high Blood Sugar levels called as IDDM.

In school, child may go for frequent urination or may not be able to see Black Board clearly or if he was very active in studies or in sports earlier, now feels lazy or tired all these symptoms are suggestive of Diabetes. He should be Investigated for Diabetes. Diabetes in children is different than from that of adults as they would need Insulin injections regularly. Junk food, chocolates, ice creams, and cold drinks have to be avoided.

B. Treatment

* Daily Insulin injection
* Diet
* Exercise

Insulin

Children are taught to take injections themselves and Blood Sugar should be monitored regularly to adjust the dose of Insulin.

Tablets are not effective and should not be given to Diabetic children.

Diet

A Diabetic child should eat small frequent meals to prevent fluctuations of the Blood Sugar.

Total calories in diet are calculated on child's age and body weight as 1000 calories at one year and additional 100 calories, food is divided in 4-6 meals.

Total calories in diet are calculated on the basis of child's age and body weight. Diet would very as per child's activity. They can have frequent meals instead of one or two big meals.

Exercise

Exercise is important for a diabetic child but, it should be avoided immediately after injection.

Diabetes-Picnic-cum-Education camps are helpful where team of Doctors, Dieticians, Diabetes educators can discuss openly with children and parents about treatment and other problems.

Counselling of parents to over come the emotional outburst of Diabetic Children is one of the important aspect of Diabetes Management.

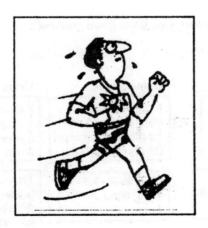

Monitoring of Diabetes
Why and How to Control?

What is Meant by Good Control?

1. Normal blood sugar levels 70 mg%-140mg%
   Acceptable for diabetics 90mg%, 180mg%
   Ideal 60-100mg% fasting, 140 mg% to 160mg% 2hrs after meals.
2. Weight—as near to ideal as possible.
3. Blood pressure normal.
4. Blood fats (Cholesterol and triglycerides) normal.
5. Glycosylated Haemoglobin levels normal.

How do you know you have good control?

By regular testing of :

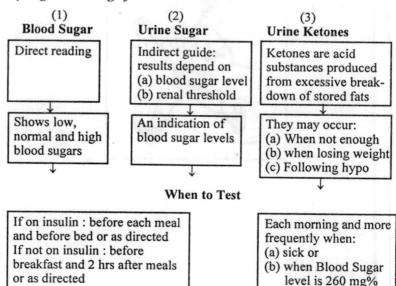

(1) **Blood Sugar**	(2) **Urine Sugar**	(3) **Urine Ketones**
Direct reading	Indirect guide: results depend on (a) blood sugar level (b) renal threshold	Ketones are acid substances produced from excessive break-down of stored fats
Shows low, normal and high blood sugars	An indication of blood sugar levels	They may occur: (a) When not enough (b) when losing weight (c) Following hypo

When to Test

If on insulin : before each meal and before bed or as directed If not on insulin : before breakfast and 2 hrs after meals or as directed	Each morning and more frequently when: (a) sick or (b) when Blood Sugar level is 260 mg% 100 ml

Also check regularly:

1. Weight.
2. Blood fats.
3. Glycosylated Heamoglobin.
4. Blood Pressure.

Why aim for good control?

1. To avoid complications:
   (a) Short-term.
   (b) Long-term affecting.
2. To lead as normal lifestyle as possible.
3. For general good health and feeling well.

How do you achieve good control?

1. Stick to your diet.
2. Get plenty of exercise.
3. Make sure your techniques are accurate.

Come to a Diabetes education programme:

4. If all these things are OK and you still have poor control than see your doctor to review your medication.

Good control of Diabetes and preventing long-term complications:

1. Diabetes may slowly damage some parts of your body. This damage can impair the quality and length of your life.
2. Certain factors may lead to the development of these complications. These are called: Risk Factors.
3. Nor everyone who has diabetes will develop complications.
4. The presence of one or more of these risk factors may increase your chance of developing the complications that are associated with diabetes.

What are the Risk Factors?

1. Poor control of Blood Sugar—Over an extended period of time.
2. Smoking—Can affect blood vessels.
3. High Blood fat levels—Can lead to damage of blood vessels.
4. High blood pressure—Can damage arteries and kidneys.

Lack of knowledge

Early warning signs may be missed. Education and early treatment my help to lesson damage.

Damage

Blood vessels		Nerves	
Large may cause build up of deposits in the vessels which can cause the blockages.	Small may cause weakness'in the vessel wall causing them to break and bleed.	Autonomic low or no response or action from the nerves controlled automatically.	Peripheral decreased sensation from the nerves to the brain.

Summary

You can decrease your risks by:

— Maintaining good control of Blood Sugar level.
— Maintaining ideal weight.
— Participating in regular exercise.
— Take medication as prescribed.
— Stop smoking.
— Participate in diabetes education programme.

Views of Diabetic Patients About their Disease

1. Diabetes is a common disease does not require any special treatment except reduction of sweet items.
2. Only 25 to 30 % of diabetic patients take regular treatment.
3. Diabetic patient consult their doctor when there is some problem like cuts at private parts (penis) or itching or for some other complications of diabetes.
4. Only 10 to 20% of diabetics get their Blood Sugar tested regularly. Majority of diabetic patients don't get their Blood Sugar tested for months together.
5. Very few diabetic patients are careful about their weight and diet control.
6. Most of the diabetic patients are eager to switch on to some magic pill after the control of their diabetes and would stop regular medicines. After few months when they go for Blood Sugar checkup they are shocked to see their very high Blood Sugar levels.
7. Diabetic patients would try to hide their reports and are not interested in discussing their problem with others.
8. Most of the diabetic patients would prefer to change the doctor who advises them to use Insulin for Blood Sugar control. They would go on changing doctors and would waste lot of time. Their reasons for refusing Insulin injections are :

- This will make habit.
- Disease has reached at its peak.
- Insulin damages body organs.

Alcohol And Diabetes

For Diabetics, is it safe to Drink?

Alcohol is every where—when the family gathers, at parties. "What will you have?" Some one asks. If you have diabetes, what do you say?

It all depends. Start by asking yourself three basic questions:

— Is my diabetes under control?
— Does my doctor agree that I am free from health problems that alcohol can make worse—for example, diabetic nerve damage or high blood pressure?
— Do I know how alcohol can affect me and my diabetes?

If you said "yes" to all three, it's okay to have an occasional drink. What does occasional mean? The American Diabetes Association suggests that you have no more than two drinks a day.

Your Body and Alcohol

Alcohol moves very quickly into the blood without being broken down (metabolized) in your stomach. Within five minutes of having a drink, there is enough alcohol in your blood to measure. Thirty to ninety minutes after having drink, the alcohol in your bloodstream is at its highest level.

Your liver does most of the job of breaking down the alcohol once it is in your body. But it needs time. If your weight is 70 kg., it will take about 2 hours to metabolize a beer or mixed drink.

If you drink alcohol faster than your liver can break it down, the excess alcohol moves through your bloodstream to other parts of your body. Brain cells are easy targets. When someone talks about getting a buzz from alcohol, this is what they are feeling.

Risks of Low Blood Glucose

If you have diabetes and take Insulin shots or oral diabetes pills, you risk low blood glucose when you drink alcohol. To protect yourself, never drink on an empty stomach. Plan to have your drink with a meal or after eating a snack that contains protein, fat or both.

How does alcohol add to your chances of having low blood glucose? It has to do with your liver.

Normally, when your blood glucose level starts to drop, your liver steps in. It goes to work changing stored carbohydrate into glucose. Then it sends the glucose out into the blood, which helps you avoid or slow down a low blood glucose reaction.

However, when alcohol enters your system, this changes. Alcohol is a toxin. Your body reacts to alcohol like a poison. The liver, wants to clear it from the blood quickly. In fact, the liver won't put out glucose again until it has taken care of the alcohol. If your blood glucose level is falling, you can quickly wind up with very low blood glucose.

This is why drinking as little as 2 ounces of alcohol (about 2 drinks) on an empty stomach can lead to very low blood glucose.

When you mix alcohol and exercise, you increase the risk of going low. This can happen because exercise helps lower your blood glucose levels. Let's say you've just played a couple of hard sets of tennis. You have a beer after the match. But in the hours after the game, your body is still working. It replaces the energy your muscles used up. To do this, it clears glucose from the blood and adds it to the muscles's store. This is why hard exercise can cause your blood glucose level to go down.

If you take Insulin or diabetes pills, they too are working to clear glucose from your blood. Unless you eat or your liver adds glucose to your blood, you could be heading for a very low blood glucose level. If you drink a beer, the alcohol will stop your liver from sending out any glucose. Your chances of going low are even greater.

If you take diabetes pills that work over a long period of ' time, such as chlorpropamide diabetese, you are at risk for very low blood glucose when drinking. This is because alcohol changes how the diabetes pill works. It makes the pill stronger and longer lasting. Hopefully, your doctor warned you about mixing long lasting diabetes pill with alcohol.

Low blood glucose when drinking is less of a risk for those with Type II diabetes who control their diabetes by diet and exercise alone. Still, alcohol is a wild card when it is mixed diet plans.

Don't Go Low

Following these guidelines to avoid low blood glucose levels when you drink:

— Never drink alcohol on an empty stomach.
— Limit yourself to 1 or 2 drinks.

If you just finished hard exercise, test your blood glucose before you drink and at least once while you're drinking. Watch for falling blood glucose levels in the hours after exercise.

Alcohol also effects your body's ability to get over a low blood glucose level. If you have low blood glucose, you may need to treat it more than once as time goes by. If you have been drinking, check your blood glucose before you go to sleep. You may need to have a snack before you retire to avoid a low blood glucose reaction while you sleep.

Heavy drinking over time can hurt your liver. It won't be able to make glucose as well. When this happens, your diabetes is harder to control.

Alcoholic drinks can have anywhere from 60 to 300 calories each.

To Eat Calories

• Put less liquor in your drink.
• Choose light beer over regular beer.
• Use dry wine.

Diabetes and Smoking

Quitting smoking is good for your diabetes. Quitting smoking is good for your health. When you quit smoking, you lower your blood glucose and blood pressure. You lower your total cholesterol, LDL cholesterol (the bad kind), and your triglycerides. When you quit smoking, you raise your HDL cholesterol (the good kind) and your oxygen intake. You even raise your life expectancy!

Quit smoking and you can reduce your risk for heart disease, blood vessel disease, kidney disease, nerve disease, dental disease, and cancer (mouth, throat, lungs, and bladder). You can reduce your risk of heart attack and stroke miscarriage or stillbirth, limited joint mobility, and colds, bronchitis, and emphysema.

Quit smoking and you can even reduce your risk for insulin resistance (when your body does not respond to insulin). No wonder people try to quit. Here are some helpful hints.

Before you Quit

- Write down each time you smoke for a week. Write down any event or activity you were doing or about to do. Save the list.
- Write down all these reasons you want to quit. Read the list each day of the week before you quit.
- Pick a day to quit and write it down. Choose a day with few pressures. That way, stress won't tempt you to smoke. You may want to do it when you've got some time off from work.
- Tell others you plan to quit. Let family, friends, and co-workers know. Seek their support. Tell them how they can help you. For example, ask them not to offer you a cigarette. Tell them what to expect when you first quit.

- Choose a method of quitting. There are many ways to quit smoking. Not every method work for every person. Your diabetes-care team may be able to help you find a method that will work for you. It might be using a nicotine patch or chewing gum. Hyposis helps some peoples stop smoking. For other, acupuncture stops the craving to smoke.
- If you would find it easier to quit with other people, think about joining a stop-smoking class.
- Practice deep breathing. Relaxation tapes may help.
- Stock up on raw vegetables and other low-fat, low-calorie snacks. Your appetite may increase after you quit smoking. You may gain weight (the average gain is 7 pounds). You may crave sweet foods.
- Begin to exercise a few weeks before you quit smoking. More activity will help you combat withdrawal symptoms and weight gain. Exercise can take the place of smoking or help you control the urge to eat. Try brisk walking, cycling, or swimming.
- Plan rewards for not smoking. For example, you might play a favourite game one week, go to a movie the next week.

After you Quit

The first 3 months or so after quitting are the hardest. Most people who return to smoking do so then. Try these tactics for staying smoke-free.

- Refer to the list you make of events or activities that were going on around the time you smoked. The next time and of those events or activities comes up, avoid it. For example, if you always smoke at happy hour, don't go.
- If you can't avoid the event, replace the cigarette with something else. Hold something else in your hand. Try a strand a beads, a polished stone, or a pen. Put something

else in your mouth, alike a toothpick. Chew gum or ice.
- If you smoke to relax, find another way to relax. Try deep breathing or relaxation exercises. If you smoke to perk up, try to walk or stretching.
- Throw away your cigarettes, butfs, lighters, matches, and ash-trays.
- Put your list or reasons for quitting where you had kept your cigarettes.
- Read your list of reasons for quitting. Remind yourself that you did not want to smoke.
- Remind yourself that all it takes is one cigarette to become a smoker again. Try to avoid even one.
- Make a list of things you like about not smoking.
- If you are worried about gaining weight, talk with your dietitian about changing your meal and exercise plans.

Vacations, Travel and Diabetes

Introduction

There is no reason for you to avoid travel just because you have diabetes. With a few extra precautions, you can take as many vacations to as many places as your imagination can suggest. A little planning and common sense are all that's required.

General Do's and Don'ts

Do carry extra supplies with you—enough to last longer than you plan to be away. That way, if you decide to extend the trip or if you are delayed, you won't have to worry about finding the supplies you need. A good rule of thumbs is to carry twice the supplies you normally need for trips of a week or less, and one week extra for longer trips.

You'll need your insulin, syringes, swabs, blood testing and urine testing equipment, some form of identification stating that you have diabetes and what your medications and dosages are. Carry extra food in case meals are delayed or missed, Don't pack these supplies in your luggage which is checked. It is safer to pack your supplies in a carry-on case.

Also Carry

- A letter and prescription from your doctor for your insulin and syringes.
- Motion sickness pills.
- Medicine to relieve possible vomiting or diarrhoea.
- Sugar cubes, dried fruit or long acting carbohydrate.
- Before you go get extra supplies of medicines.
- See your doctor.

Travelling by Car

Auto trips can be very enjoyable. But a long drive could leave you miles from available food at your scheduled meal times, so bring along a snack to sandwiches long as it's enough to fill the needs of your individual meal plan. Then, even if you have car trouble, you won't take the chance of missing a meal.

If you're doing the driving be sure you have about 15 grams of carbohydrate every hour to guard against low blood sugar and a possible Insulin reaction which could affect your driving ability. A small piece of fruit such as a peach, pear, apple or orange, two large sugar cubes, a small box of raisins, or two crackers will provide about the right amount of carbohydrate. Also, don't forget the importance of blood testing during the trip to keep a close watch on blood glucose levels.

Don't keep your Insulin anywhere in the car where it could become very hot or cold, such as the dashboard or boot. Extreme temperatures can change your insulin's effectiveness. A good rule of thumb: if the temperature is comfortable for you, it is a safe temperature for your Insulin.

Buses and Trains

When you travel by bus or train, rest stops and meal times may not match your schedule. And there can be unexpected delays. Carry a snack such as packaged cheese and crackers, or a sandwich, or a piece of fruit, so that you can provide your body with the sugar it needs at your regular meal-time. And, of course, carry your insulin, syringes, and diabetes identifications with you, rather than leaving those things with your luggage. If you're travelling alone, it's a good idea to let the driver or conductor know that you have diabetes, just in case you should have a problem.

In flight Injections

On a long flight, you may be scheduled for an injection while you're in the air. Follow your normal procedure with one difference put only one half as much air into your Insulin bottle as you normally would. Cabin pressure in high-altitude flight is lower than pressure on the ground, so you won't need as much. pressure inside the bottle to balance the Insulin you draw.

Carry a Sugar Source

You should always carry some form of sugar that can be eaten easily. This could be food such as raisins, sugar cubes or a piece of fresh fruit. Any of these sources can give you enough sugar to help you avoid a low blood sugar reaction (also called an "Insulin reaction" or "hypoglycaemia").

When you are travelling chances are your routine will be different from when you are at home, and the risks of a reaction are greater. Even people who normally very aware of the signs of a reaction can be caught off guard by the stress and excitement of travel.

Your doctor may suggest one of the instant glucose preparations. These are designed to be given by mouth, and to get sugar into your bloodstream quickly in case of emergency. If your doctor does suggest one of these preparations, make sure that someone you're travelling with understands how to use it.

Blood Testing is a Must

The excitement and stress of a vacation, the changes in your daily routine, meal timing, and the kinds of food available can all affect your blood sugar levels. Test your blood for sugar at least times.

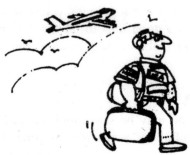

Are You Losing Weight

One has to keep the weight under control for proper Diabetes Management. If persons is over weight obese he develops Insulin resistance. *Efficacy* of Insulins actions or tissues is reduced and Diabetes becomes uncontrolled. Sometimes Diabetic patients go on losing weight inspite of regular treatment. The reasons may be:

1. Either you are taking very low calories diet in place of diet advised to you by your doctor (say you are advised to take 1800 calories diet buy you are taking 1200 calories diet).

2. Whenever sugar levels are very high and diabetes is uncontrolled one is passing sugar with urine. For Energy sugar is not available, it uses available sugar in body and thereby causing weight loss.

3. When patient is using medicines like Metformin, Glyciphage, Glycomet or Capsule DBI-TD etc. These medicines reduce appetite and reduce weight.

4. If there are associated diseases like Tuberculosis, Thyroid disease *or* patient is having loose motions or vomiting.

Treatment

If even with balanced diet patient is losing weight then it is matter of concern and he/she should consult doctor.

— Have proper calories diet consult dietician/doctor.
— Don't adjust/change medicines yourself.
— If your doctor advises you to take Insulin Don't Resist.

It will stop weight loss and would control Blood Sugar.

Diabetes Prevention and High Risk Group to Develop Diabetes

Incidence of diabetes is increasing more and more, new cases are detected everyday due to public awareness, at the same time everyone ask this question: How we can prevent Diabetes and its complications?

One thing is sure that NIDDM can be prevented, its onset can be delayed and one can even prevent complications to great extent.

Change in lifestyle, food habits and sedentary habits have contributed to this increase in the incidence of Diabetes.

IDDM—Disease presents in childhood, islet cell antibodies and insulin auto-antibodies are present at the age of 2 years—By some virus infection or other factors cause activation of Immune response—this in turn destroy Beta-cells of Pancrease.

Screening can be done by analysing genetic factors and Immune measures marriage between two diabetics should be avoided.

In NIDDIM

It takes about 10-15 years to develop symptoms of diabetes. During this period initially there is impaired Glucose tolerance test then abnormal glucose tolerance test and finally Symptomatic diabetes. As this problem is seen in relatives of NIDDM thorough screening of family members for impaired/Abnormal glucose tolerance test can detect potential future diabetic patients. Regular exercise, weight reduction and diet control can stop the progression of disease—and delay the symptoms for many years. Antioxidants should be taken regularly.

Marriage of two diabetics should be avoided.

Diabetes and Depression

Major depressive disorder is present in 15 to 20% of patients with diabetes. Even after successful treatment depression will return in 80% of diabetic patients.

Depression in diabetes has a special relevance, as depression has association with poor compliance with diabetic treatment, poor glycaemic control and increased risk for micro and macrovascular complications.

Type II diabetes one hundred and eighty-eight patients between 40-47 years were studied for symptoms and well being in relation to glycaemic control.

Higher HbA_{1c} levels were significantly associated with higher symptoms scores (Total score hyperglycaemic and neuropathic score) with worse mood (total score, displeasure score, depression, tension, fatigue) and the worse general well being.

The data suggested that better glycaemic control in Type II diabetes is associated with fewer Physical Symptoms, better mood and better well being in non-hypoglycaemic HbA_{1c} range.

"Diabetes is associated with increased risk of psychological disturbance especially for those with more diabetes related complications."

Insulin dependent diabetic patients who reported feeling depressed, anxious or stressed out were among least likely to successfully lower their Blood Sugar Levels even after learning to practice relaxation techniques.

Aspirin for Diabetics

Diabetics have as 2-4 fold increase in the risk of dying from the complications of heart diseases.

American Diabetes Association Recommends use of Asprin for both primary prevention and secondary prevention.

Primary Prevention

Use of Asprin in High Risk people with diabetes would prevent them from heart attacks and stroke.

Risk Factors in Type I and II Diabetes are:

- A Family History of Heart Attacks
- Cigarette Smoking
- Hypertenion
- Obesity
- Albminuria
- People with High Cholesterol and Triglyceride levels
- Those who are above 30 years

All these people can take tablet of Asprin as per recommendation of their doctor. You must consult your Doctor before using Asprin.

Always take Asprin after Food.

Use of Asprin for Secondary Prevention

Your Doctor would recommend you to take Asprin if you have evidence of large vessel disease, i.e.,

(i) After MYOCARDIAL INFRACTION (Heart Attack)
(ii) After By-pass Surgery
(iii) After Stroke

(iv) Evidence of having Blockage of Arteries of leg

(v) Those who have ANGINA.

Therefore use of Asprin is recommended for both, i.e.

(i) Those who are going to develop complications and for

(ii) Those who already have evidence of complications and to prevent further recurrence.

Are You in High Risk Group
for Diabetes

Please reply all Questions

1.	Are you overweight? (this obesity is Apple Type)	Yes/No.
2.	Are you Leading Sedantry Lifestyle. (No Exercise)?	Yes/No.
3.	Do you have Family History of Diabetes?	Yes/No.
4.	Are you over 40 years of Age?	Yes/No.
5.	Did you have Diabetes during Pregnancy?	Yes/No.
6.	Do you suffer from High Blood Pressure?	Yes/No.
7.	Do you have High Blood Cholesterol and Triglycerides in your Blood?	Yes/No.

If your answer is yes to any of the above question you are in a high risk group for development of Diabetes.

Diabetes can be prevented

If you are in high risk group get (G.T.T.), Glucose Tolerance Test. If it is Abnormal then control your diet, reduce weight by regular exercise. You can prevent diabetes by these means.

People who carry more weight on the hips and thighs are pear-shaped. People who carry more weight around the waist and abdomen are apple-shaped. Apple-shaped people are more likely to have blood vessel disease, heart disease, high blood pressure, high blood fat levels, insulin resistance, and poor blood glucose control.

My Story of Diabetes

Hypoglycaemic Story

Mrs. Goel aged 40 years was brought to hospital emergency at 6 a.m., she was unconscious at that time. Relatives gave the history that she is a Diabetic patient and was on Insulin injections. Her hand and feet were cold and clothes were wet. She would have headache in the morning and disturbed sleep. Her Blood Sugar was 45 mg/100ml. She was given I.V. glucose in hospital and within 1/2 an hour started recovering. She recovered completely after 4 hours. According to her she missed her evening meals after Insulin injection in morning (long acting). This was Hypoglycaemic Coma occurs due to sudden decrease in Blood Sugar after Insulin or tablets. After tablets specially this low Blood Sugar state can last up to 72 years.

Second Story

Till 1976 I was alright, then I started having cuts and itching around penis. I consulted doctor who advised Blood Sugar testing which revealed Diabetes. I was advised to take certain pills and in this way 16 years passed away.

In 1992, I sustained some injury to feet and was showing to my General Physician who would do dressing of wound. One day I noticed black colour at the injury site and showed it to Diabetologist. It was gangrene of great toe and my toe was (amputated) removed. I was able to walk again.

In between I used to have chest discomfort and high blood pressure and was taking medicines for it too.

In 1992 December as soon as finished my dinner, some labourers who were working in home called me from down stairs. I immediately started coming down but on the way I felt short of breath and suffocation in chest. I was shifted to hospital and to my surprise it was heart attack, not a gas discomfort or indigestion which I was thinking. Now I have undergone By-pass Surgery and on regular Insulin injections.

IDDIM Story

I am 13 year old boy and taking Insulin injections regularly.

I was alright till the age of 9 years and then had viral fever. I was diagnosed having Pneumonia and at the same time having diabetes. No one was ready to accept it, they attributed it to antibiotics or treatment. Before this attack I used to feel weakness I would feel extreme weakness and sleepy but my parents thought that this was due to my excessive play and physical activities. Finally, I landed in hospital both with chest infection and at that time I was diagnosed having Diabetes which would require regular Insulin injections.

Now I take injection twice daily and feel like any other child except having daily pricks.

My Experience

I am a Diabetic child. When I returned from the hospital 3 years before it was very difficult for my relatives or society to accept that I am a Diabetic. They considered Diabetes is a cure. (मधुमेह एक अभिशाप है।) I would have felt very sad that I am not a normal child, but my family gave me strength to fight with Diabetes. I accepted Diabetes in my life as a challenge. I want to give as assurance to my society that I am like a normal child. I can do everything what a non-Diabetic do. Only I have to take some precautions. Even Diabetic person can live healthy life as compared to normal person. Why our society considered Diabetes a problem? They considered taking injections twice a day is a very big problem. We eat food, drink waters, go to school, board bus, drive car/scooter and do many scores of other activities. Even we breath every second. Do we consider all these activities as a problem? Friends let us take a pledge and consider ourselves not a symbol of sympathy and do not avail of any special privileged offered. Behave like a normal child and do all that is expected of a normal child. Someone has rightly said that—

Diabetic Life is a challenge	Meet it
Diabetic Life is a Struggle	Accept it
Diabetic Life is a Battle	Fight it
Diabetic Life is a Problem	Solve it
Diabetic Life is a Sorrow	Overcome it
Diabetic Life is a Game	Play it

—Bhawna Chawla, XII Class (16 years)

Hall leads Hopes in 100ml Freestyle

Gary Hall will try to give the USA the lift it needs in the 100-metre freestyle in the Sydney Olympics.

Hall, 25, saved the USA from its first loss in Olympics history in the 4 × 100 freestyle relay at the 1996 Atlanta Game. Swimming the anchor leg, he produced what was then the fastest relay split ever (47.45 seconds) and brought the USA from third to first, winning in a Olympic record of 3.15.41 minutes. He also won silver in the individual 100, just 0.26 seconds behind Alexander Popov of Russia.

Hall was diagnosed with diabetes, and he thought his career was over. He learned to manage his diabetes by constantly monitoring his Blood Sugar, balancing his energy expenditure with his eating and taking appropriate medication.

The thing is every time he wins a race, it is a victory against diabetes—a hope for millions of sufferers wanting to lead not just normal but winning lives.

Foot Care in Diabetes

As the sensations of pain and temperature are diminished in feet due to involvement of nerves in diabetes and one should be very careful. If there is some cut or ulcer due to shoe bite Diabetic patient will notice it very late.

Each day, set aside a regular time (such as after bathing) to inspect your feet. Check between your toes as well as all the sides for blisters, cuts, scratches, cracks, corns, and calluses. Examine the balls of your feet for dryness and broken skin. During examination, look or feel for warts and ingeowth toe nails.

If you notice anything unusual—particularly sores, redness, or infection—see your doctor at once.

Foot Care Do's

* Keep feet clean, warm and dry.
* Wash (Don't soak) feet daily with warm (not hot) water.
* Use mild hand soap; rinse well.
* Dry feet thoroughly, especially between toes.
* Powder feet and shoes after bathing.
* Use mild lubricating lotion in small amounts and massage well (between toes).
* Trim toe nails straight across; file with emery board.
* Wear comfortable, well-fitting shoes (leather is best).
* Break in new shoes gradually.
* Inspect shoes for objects, torn lining, rough spots which can injure feet.
* Wear clean socks everyday.
* Check socks or stockings for drainage or unusual odour.
* Wear loose-fitting socks to bed if needed to protect from cold.

For proper foot care, what you don't do is sometimes just as important as what you do. Here are some general "to-dos" that, with daily attention, will become second nature.

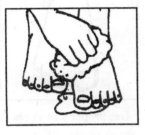

Wash feet with water and soap

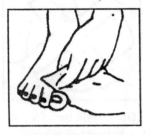

Clean the area between two toes

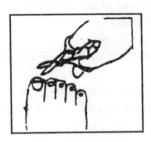

Cut nails properly

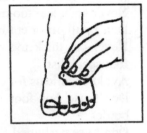

Use moisture for skin

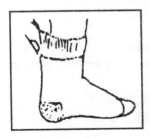

Use clean and proper size socks and stockings

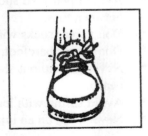

Keep your foot dry and warm

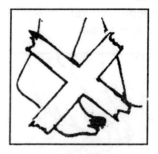

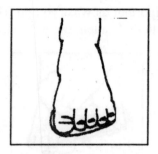

Don't walk bare footed   Use proper size shoes
in home or outside

Foot Care Don'ts

*   Avoid exposure of feet to extremes of hot and cold.
*   Never keep feet too moist or too dry.
*   Don't pull off or cut loose pieces of skin.
*   Never cut thick toe nails, corns, or calluses. Rely on a foot specialist.
*   Avoid chemicals for corns or callus removal.
*   Don't use hot foot soaks, heating pads, or hot-water bottles.
*   Don't use perfumed lotions.
*   Don't use adhesive tape on skin.
*   Don't wear shoes without stockings or socks.
*   Avoid open-toed shoes, particularly sandals with thongs between toes.
*   Don't wear socks with holes.
*   Don't walk barefoot, even indoors.
*   Never go without shoes around a swimming pool or hot beach.
*   Avoid sitting with legs crossed.
*   Never walk on an injured foot.

HbA$_{1C}$ and Mean Blood Glucose (Over a period of 8-10 weeks) and Other Tests

Diabetes is a chronic, yet treatable condition. Recent studies have shown the value of light blood sugar control in delaying diabetic complications. Good blood sugar control is beneficial for all people with diabetes.

Uncontrolled Diabetes over a period of time leads to following complication:

1. Eye problems
2. Heart Attack
3. Kidney diseases
4. Nerve damage

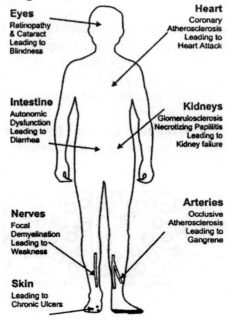

Eyes
Retinopathy & Cataract Leading to Blindness

Heart
Coronary Atherosclerosis Leading to Heart Attack

Intestine
Autonomic Dysfunction Leading to Diarrhea

Kidneys
Glomerulosclerosis Necrotizing Papillitis Leading to Kidney failure

Arteries
Occlusive Atherosclerosis Leading to Gangrene

Nerves
Focal Demyelination Leading to Weakness

Skin
Leading to Chronic Ulcers

Suggested Investigations

Following investigations should be done to keep a check complications.

Frequency	Investigations
Every fortnight	Fasting & PP Glucose (Post Breakfast and Lunch)
Every 3 months	HBA_{IC} and MBG
Every year	Urea, Uric Acid, Creatinine, Lipid Profile, HBA_{IC} and MBG, Micro-albuminuria and Urine Routine

Of these two main tests related to help achieve good blood sugar control are:

1. Blood glucose level monitoring
2. HBA_{IC} and Mean Blood Glucose (MBG)

What is HBA_{IC}?

In the blood stream, sticky glucose attaches to hemoglobin (hemoglobin is the protein in red blood cells that carries oxygen). As the glucose level increases, so does the amount of hemoglobin with glucose riding piggyback. Once glucose attaches to hemoglobin, it stays attached and becomes glychemoglobin-HBA_{IC}.

The HBA_{IC} test is a with a money. It tells your doctor about average glucose control over the past 8-10 weeks.

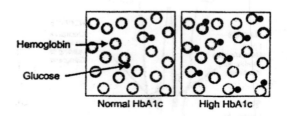

Normal HbA1c   High HbA1c

Benefits of HbA$_{IC}$ Testing

By measuring the percentage of HBA$_{IC}$, doctors can estimate the average glucose level over the life span of the red blood cells. In other words, the HBA$_{IC}$ test reveals long-term control over the last 8-10 weeks.

HBA$_{IC}$ test values will begin to reflect major changes in diet and therapy in about 3 to 4 weeks after the change.

While blood sugar testing is like a snap shot, HBA$_{IC}$ testing is more like a full-length movie—it provides an overall view of your glucose control.

Reaching Your Target

Your doctor uses your HBA$_{IC}$ results to fine-tune your treatment. The normal range for the HBA$_{IC}$ test is between .4% and 6%. However, people with diabetes may have an HBA$_{IC}$ level greater than 8%. In uncontrolled diabetes, the level may be higher. The ADA recommends that the target for good glucose control is 7% HBA$_{IC}$.

How often should you be tested for HBA$_{IC}$?

Getting an HBA$_{IC}$ test is easy. It only requires one sample of blood, drawn at anytime of the day, including right after a meal.

Frequency	Condition
Twice a year	If your have stable glucose control and are meeting your treatment targets.
Every 3 Months	If your treatment changes or you are not meeting your targets.

To ensure the best possible care, be sure to ask your doctor for an HBA$_{IC}$ test today. Also, it is important to ensure that your doctor uses a certified HBA$_{IC}$ test. Remember, you'll be looking at the trend in your HBA$_{IC}$ numbers over time, so quality is important.

Using Your HbA$_{IC}$ Test Results

If your HBA$_{IC}$ level is less than 7% you are doing an excellent job of obtaining near normal glucose levels.

If your HBA$_{IC}$ level is greater than 8%, some change in your treatment plan may be needed; check with your doctor.

Achieving your target HBA$_{IC}$ level is the best way to reduce the risk of developing long-term complications.

Get Your Pipes Checked

It is a good idea to get pipes checked. In people with long standing and poorly controlled diabetes, high blood glucose can effect the small blood vessels supplying the kidney and retina and large blood vessels supplying the Brain, Heart and lower limbs (legs and feet). Narrowing of arteries is a normal part of growing old but it is more common in people who have diabetes. Smoking and poor diabetes control make it worse, if you get pain in calf and foot on walking it indicates that the blood supply to the legs is insufficient and that there is obstruction to the blood flow. It can even lead to gangrene which may require amputation of foot or leg.

If you have any of the symptoms listed, check with your doctor to see if you should schedule a painless vascular examination. Early detection of vascular problems can help you to *avoid serious complications and help you enjoy your life to the fullest.*

Current Symptoms:

*   Claudication Rt ☐ Lt ☐
  (leg pain during walking which disappears with rest)   ☐
*   Limb hair loss/Absence   ☐
*   Skin colour changes   ☐
*   Trophic Nails   ☐
*   Numbness, Tingling   ☐
*   Cold Hands or Feet   ☐
*   Extermity weakness   ☐
*   Ulcerations   ☐

Care of Kidney in Diabetes

Micral Test (Test for Micro-Albuminurea)

This Test detects microscopic amounts of albumin in the urine and signifies signs of very early kidney damage.

In the early stage of kidney damage, there is a leak of very small amounts of protein (albumin) into the urine. If it is a consistent finding, it indicates that your kidneys have been damaged by your diabetes. If this is the case, then attention to the control of your blood glucose and treatment of high blood pressure is of great importance, as this can stabilize or even reverse the condition.

Test is very simple and for this we only need a sample of urine.

Correlation Between HBA$_{IC}$ and Glucose Levels

HbA$_{IC}$% Gloucose	Mean Blood mg/dl
4	65
5	100
6	135
7	170
8	205
9	240
10	275
11	310
12	345

Self-Evaluation About Diabetes Control

You read the Questionnaire and judge yourself about:

1. Do you Keep records of Blood Glucose Tests or Urine-Tests? **Yes/No**
2. Have your ever adjusted dose of Insulin or Tablets by seeing your records? **Yes/No**
3. At hotels or restaurants you were able to decide the food of your choice according to need of calories prescribed for you? **Yes/No**
4. Have you even experienced symptoms of hypoglycaemia or low Blood Sugar with your regular exercise programme and again have you adjusted the dose of insulin or oral medicines? **Yes/No**
5. Have you actively participated in the learning process, i.e. group discussions and attending lecture? **Yes/No**
6. Were you able to manage Diabetes during stressful situations, i.e. emotional upset or during some infection etc.? **Yes/No**
7. Have you ever given up treatment schedule thinking it is futile or useless? **Yes/No**
8. Do you believe that Home Blood glucose home monitoring (HBGM) is helpful for better living? **Yes/No**
9. Do you think that sharing the views of diabetics who have lived and coped diabetes for many years, are useful? **Yes/No**
10. Have you ever indulged in excessive drinking knowing that this would have adverse affect on your diabetes control? **Yes/No**

Score

A. If you have score of
   8 Yes
   2 No
   Then you are having excellent understanding of Diabetes and you can manage your Diabetes.

B. If you have score of
   6 Yes
   4 No
   Although you know about Diabetes, still it needs proper attention to prevent complications of Diabetes.

C. If your score is
   4 Yes or Less
   Then you are having poor control of Diabetes. You are the one who is prone to develop complications of Diabetes. You need proper counselling.

Questions Diabetic Patient Usually Ask

1. Q Whether my disease will be cured or not?
   A Diabetes is a disease which can be controlled by regular exercise, diet control, by oral medicines or by Insulin injections.

2. Q What about sweets and fruits?
   A You can eat fruits and sweets but adjust the food. Say today you want to take one slice of mango, you should not take other fruits on that day.

3. Q Can I substitute extra one tablet for ice-creams or extra diet?
   A No. One should avoid it as it will disturb your diabetes control. Never take medicines along with alcohol.

4. Q If I have forgotten to take Insulin in the morning, can I take double dose in the evening?
   A No. One might go in to hypoglycaemia.

5. Q Is it true that heart attack is without pain in diabetics. Then how it is diagnosed?
   A Heart attack is painless or silent. Usually there is no pain; patient gets breathlessness and checking sensations. E.C.G. helps in diagnosis.

6. Q Is it true that once Insulin started it is for ever?
   A If your Blood Sugar levels are very high and not coming under control with medicines your doctor my advise you to take Insulin. Once Blood Sugar starts coming down then Insulin can be withdrawn.

7. Q Is there any test which one can find out whether kidney's are affected or not?
   A Yes. Kidney's are involved in diabetes invariably. It depends upon duration of diabetes and raised Blood

Sugar Levels. Earliest manifestation is appearances of proteins, called albumin in urine. It takes about 5 to 10 years from this stage to reach the final stage of end stage kidney failure. If one keeps Blood Sugar and blood pressure under control at this stage, this process can be reversed.

8. Q   Please explain sexual relationship with diabetes control?

    A   Uncontrolled Diabetes leads to sexual weakness, and impotence and instead of trying sexual stimulants or alcohol one should try to control Blood Sugar. It is true that persistent, high Blood Sugar would worsen the situation. There is urge but you can't perform.

Important Points to Remember

1. If Parents are Diabetic then you have to be careful regarding your weight because as soon as you cross 40 years of age and if you are obese/over weight by 40% you are prone to develop Diabetes. So keep your weight under control.
2. Regular Exercise and Balanced diet will keep your Diabetes under control.
3. Don't change the tablets which you are taking for the control of Diabetes on other advice and don't take these tablets with alcohol.
4. Diabetics who smoke are the worst sufferers.
5. Don't substitute extra tablet for your extra food/ice cream.
6. Never stop your treatment by reading any advertisement in Newspaper for any magic medicine. You may disturb your well control disease by stopping treatment.
7. Avoid Sex therapies as all such treatment will not improve sexual performance until and unless your Diabetes is under control.
8. To improve the quality of life if you are advised Insulin treatment, it does not mean that your disease has reached at its end.
9. Don't stop your medication without doctor's advice.

Diabetes Care During Other Infections

When you get sick like have cold and cough, stomach upset, loose motions you may not be able to take your usual insulin or diabetes medicines as you normally take. You may not feel like eating. During this period blood sugar levels may go up or down.

What About Medicine Dosage

One should never stop taking medicine during this period. You may need extra dosage to control infection during certain infections when you are not able to take oral medicine your doctor would like to put you on regular insulins. This may be for limited period but essential to control infection.

If blood sugar is high, infections also (Flareup) Become difficult to control. We have to control both infection and blood sugar same time.

Cough syrups, and Decongestants increase blood sugar. Asprin, crocin, some antibiotics may lower your blood glucose levels.

How About Food

You can eat your normal diet, sometimes semi-solids like Khichri (Rice+dal), *Daliya* (OAT). But consume plenty of liquids. If you have diarrhoea then take cup of fluid each hour.

You can use sugar free tea, coffee, lemon + salt in water. You can have fruit juices which have 15gm carbohydrate.

Blood Sugar Testing

Because of infections, and release of more hormones during this time sugar levels fluctuates it is better to check your blood sugar level more often. Urine examination for ketones will help to rule out very high level of sugar.

Contact your Doctor

*   If you are sick for more than 3-4 days.
*   If you are having vomiting and loose motions.
*   If blood sugar is above 250 mg/dl.
*   If urine is showing ketones.
*   If you have chest pain, breathing difficulty, fruity breath and dry tongue.

Timely help from doctor can help you to recover early.

Insulin Pumps

Insulin Pump is newer method of delivery of insulin in body by battery powered computerized device. Its size is about the size of mobile phone. Inside the pump is syringe which have short acting insulin with a gear driven plunger. A tube is attached to the pump and other end is attached with the needle or catheter which is inserted in the skin of abdomen or thigh and insulin is delivered through this into body.

Benefits

*   Blood Glucose level remain near normal
*   If you have marred fluctuations this will help you top smooth them out.
*   You can adjust dose as per requirement of body.

Problems

*   Biggest problem is cost of pump.
*   *Infection* : Place where your body enters become infected always clean the area before you insert the needle by proper antibiotic lotion or cream.
*   *Ketoacidosis*: Sometimes tube can get block then sugar level may go high and person can develop diabetic ketoacidosis. Best way to protect is do frequent blood sugar monitoring.

Stress and Diabetes

Our lives are full of factors that can cause stress. Stress can be physical or an illness stress can be mental, like job related marriage, etc. Good or bad stress which lasts longer affects your body. Diabetes is a physical stress. That lasts a long time.

During stress, hormones are pumped into your blood which in turn release stored blood glucose and stored fat for extra energy. This extra energy helps to face this stress.

In diabetic patients as there is not enough insulin, glucose and fat levels increase in the blood and this can lead to high blood sugar levels and high ketones.

Physical stress causes blood glucose levels to go up in most people with diabetes. Mental stress can influence in both ways—may cause blood sugar levels to go up and in some may lower.

How to Handle Stress

1. Make lists of things that stress you.
2. Learn how you react to stress. You may feel tense, anxious, upset, or angry. You may feel tired, sad, or empty. You may have stomach up set or headache.
3. Change your reaction you can't stop things that cause stress. But you can change how you react. If you feel stressed try following tactics.

1. *Breathe Deeply*. This is called as *Sudershan kirya* too. You sit or lie down. Close your eyes. Breathe in deeply and slowly. Let all the breathe out. Breathe in and out again (for 15 to 20 times). Start to relax your muscles. Do it twice in a day.

* Lie Down : Lie down close your eyes tense and relax the muscles of each part or body from head to feet.

* Loosen up and shake parts of body.
* Get a massage.
* Think about good things and talk about your troubles with family members or friends. Put your problems on paper.
* Stay active and listen to music you may find it soothing.
* Say no if you don't like anything.
* Have a hearty healthy laugh.
* Eat Wisely. During stress you may need more vitamins, protein and minerals. Eat, fruits like oranges, nuts, seeds, and beans, chicken, fish and egg white.
  For minerals :- low fat milk, curd and cheese.
* Get 6-8 hours of sleep a day.

Diet During Illness

If you feel ill or are unable to have your usual meals, it is important to:

1. Have your usual dose of Insulin or tablets at your normal time.

2. If you are too sick to eat your usual diet, you must substitute suitable food or fluids for the carbohydrate exchanges in your diet.

   Try some of the alternatives given below.

   Each one of the following is approximately 1 Carbohydrate Exchange

150-200ml	Fruit juice
150 ml	Ordinary lemonade/ordinary soft drink
1/2 cup	Ordinary Jelly
7	Jelly beans
2 or 3	Dry biscuits
2 scoops	Ice cream

3. If you are vomiting or have diarrhoea, the risk of hypoglycaemia and dehydration will be greatly reduced if you take small amounts of sugar containing fluids every 30 minutes, e.g. 1/2 cup of ordinary lemonade.

   Plenty of additional fluid is also advisable.

   If your Blood Sugar Levels are persistently above 270 mg% joule/diet fluids only (e.g. clear broths, water, diet soft drinks and diet cordial).

4. Test your Blood Sugar level more frequently, perhaps every hour, and test your urine for ketone.

Remember :

* Take your usual Insulin or tablets
* Test Blood Sugar Levels more frequently
* Test for ketones
* Call your doctor

Foods Can be Used Freely

The following foods may be used freely to increase the variety in your meals.

Vegetables	—	All vegetables except potato, corn and legumes.
Fruits	—	lemon lime, Malta/Grape fruit, small quantities of watermelon, Guava and berries. One apple or two oranges or two slices of Papaya or Guava or combination of above in small amount can be taken.
Beverages	—	Tea, coffee, soda and plain mineral water, clear soups/broth.
Miscellaneous	—	Herbs and spices, garlic, ginger, mustard, chilli powder, curry paste and powder, vinegar, no oil dressings, tomato paste, tomato puree, essences such as vanilla, lemon and peppermint, cocoa.
Use Sparingly (as high in salt)	—	Meat and fish pastes.

Acceptable Special Diet Foods

    —   Artificial sweetners (liquid, powder, tablets)
           Aspartame (Nutrasweet)
           Saccharine, Cyclamate
           Acesulphame K, Sucralose (Splenda)
           Isomalt, maltodextrin, polydextrose
    —   **Products**
           Low joule or diet jellies

Low joule jams
Low joule or diet cordials
Low joule or diet soft drinks
Diet topping
Sugarless chewing gum

Note: During pregnancy, Aspartame or Acesulphame K in small amounts are the preferred artificial sweetners.

Diet Charts

These Diet Charts are according to food habits of different regions of India—North India or South India

Diet Chart for Over Weight and Obese (Fat) Persons

1200 Calories

Sample Menu

	North	South	East	West
Pre-breakfast	1 tea without Sugar 4 Marie biscuits 1/2 apple orange	1 coffee without sugar 3 banana chips biscuits 1/2 apple	1 tea without sugar 4 Marie biscuits 1/2 small	1 coffee or tea without sugar 4 Marie biscuits 1/2 apple
Breakfast	2 slices bread 1 glass skimmed milk 1 egg	2 Idlies with chutney 1 glass skimmed milk 1 egg	2 slices bread 1 glass skimmed milk 1 egg	2 slices bread 1 glass skimmed milk 1 egg
Lunch	3 Chapaties 1/2 Katori vegetable 1 teaspoon oil for cooking 2/3 glass curd	2 katories rice 1/4 Katori sambar 1 teaspoon oil for cooking 2/3 glass curd	2 Katories rice 1/2 Katori vegetable 1 teaspoon oil for cooking 2/3 glass curd	1 1/2 chapaties and 1 katorie rice 1/2 Katori vegetable 1 teaspoon oil for cooking 2/3 glass curd
Evening snack	1 tea without sugar 2 Monaco biscuits 1/2 apple	1 coffee without sugar 2 Monaco biscuits 1/2 orange	1 tea without sugar 2 Monaco biscuits 1 piece papaya	1 coffee or tea without sugar 2 Monaco biscuits 1/2 apple

Dinner

2 Chapaties	1 Katories rice+	2 katories rice	1 1/2 chapaties
	1 1/2 chapaties	and 1 katori rice	
1 Katori	1 Katori sambar	1 katori	1 Katori
vegetable		vegetable	vegetable
1 teaspoon oil	1 teaspoon oil	1teaspoon oil	1 teaspoon oil
for cooking	for cooking	for cooking	for cooking
1/3 glass curd	1/3 glass curd	1/3 glass curd	1/3glass curd
1/2 katori	1/2 katori lentils	1/2 katori	1/2 katori
Rajmah		lentils	lentiles

Diet Chart for Overweight and Obese Persons

1400 calories

Sample Menu

	North	South	East	West
Pre-breakfast				
	1tea without sugar	1 coffee without sugar	1 tea without sugar	1 coffee or tea without sugar
	4 Marie biscuits	3 banana chips biscuits	4 Marie biscuits	4 Marie biscuits
	1/2 apple or orange	1/2 apple	1/2 small orance	1/2 apple
Breakfast				
	3 slices bread	3Idlies with chutney	3 slices bread	3 slices bread
	1 teaspoon butter	1 teaspoon oil for cooking	1 teaspoon oil for cooking	1 teaspoon oil for cooking
	1 glass skimmed milk	1 glass skimmed milk	1 glass skimmed milk	1 glass skimmed milk
	1 egg	1 egg	1 egg	1 egg
Lunch				
	3 Chapaties	2 katories rice	2 Katories rice	1 1/2 chapaties and 1 katories rice
	1/2 Katori vegetable	1/2 katori sambar	1katori vegetable	1 Katori vegetable
	1 teaspoon oil for cooking	1 teaspoon oil for cooking	1 teaspoon oil for cooking	1 teaspoon oil for cooking
	1/3 glass curd	1/3 glass curd	1/3 glass curd	1/3 glass curd
	1/2 Katori Rajmah	1/2 kator Lentils	1/2 Katori Lentils	1/2 Katori Lentils

Evening snack

1 tea without sugar	1 coffee without sugar	1 tea without sugar	1 coffee or tea without sugar
2 Monaco biscuits	2 Monaco biscuits	2 Monaco biscuits	2Monaco biscuits
1/2 apple	1/2 orange	1 piece papaya	1/2 apple

Dinner

2 Chapaties	1 Katori rice+ 1-1/2 chapaties	2 katories rice	1-1/2 chapaties and 1 katori rice
1/2 Katori vegetable	1/2 Katori sambar	1/2 katori vegetable	1/2 Katori vegetable
2/3glass curd	1/3glass curd	1/3glass curd	1/3glass curd
1 teaspoon oil for cooking	1 teaspoon oil for cooking	1teaspoon oil for cooking	1 teaspoon oil for cooking
1 piece chicken breast	1 piece chicken breast	1 piece fish	1 piece chicken breast

Diet Chart for Persons Working in Office, Doctors, Business Food Chart according to different regions of India

1800 calories

Sample Menu

	North	South	East	West
Pre-breakfast	1tea without Sugar	1 coffee without sugar	1tea without sugar	1 coffee or tea without sugar
	4 Monaco biscuits	6 banana chips biscuits	4 Monaco biscuits	4 Monaco biscuits
	1/2 apple	1/2 small apple	1/2 small orange	1/2 apple
Breakfast	4 slice bread	4 Idlies with chutney	4 slices bread	4 slices bread
	1teaspoon butter	1 teaspoon oil for cooking	1 teaspoon oil for cooking	1 teaspoon butter for cooking
	1 glass skimmed milk	1 glass skimmed milk	1 glass skimmed milk	1 glass skimmed milk
	1 egg	1 egg	1 egg	1 egg

Lunch

3 Chapaties	2 katories rice	2 Katories rice	1-1/2 chapaties and 1 katori rice
1 Katori vegetable	1/2 katori sambar	1 katorie vegetable	1 Katorie vegetable
1-1/2 teaspoon oil for cooking	1-1/2 teaspoon oil for cooking	1-1/2 teaspoon oil for cooking	1-1/2teaspoon oil for cooking
2/3 glass curd	2/3 glass curd	2/3 glass curd	2/3 glass curd
3/4 Katori Rajmah	3/4 katori Lentils	3/4 Katori Lentils	3/4 Katori Lentils

Evening snack

1 tea without sugar	1 coffee without sugar	1 tea without sugar	1 coffee or tea without sugar
8 Maire biscuits	8 Maire biscuits	8 Maire biscuits	8 Maire biscuits
1/2 apple	1/2 orange	2 piece papaya	1/2 apple

Dinner

3 Chapaties+1 katori rice	2Katories rice+ 1-1/2 chapaties	3katories rice &2 chapaties	1-1/2 chapaties
1Katori vegetable	1Katori vegetable	1katori vegetable	1Katori vegetable
1-1/2 teaspoon oil for cooking	1-1/2 teaspoon oil for cooking	1-1/2 teaspoon oil for cooking	1-1/2 teaspoon oil for cooking
1/3 glass curd	1/3 glass curd	1/3 glass curd	1/3 glass curd
1 piece chicken	1 piece chicken	1 piece fish	1 piece chicken

The vegetables may be used as desired. Carbohydrates and calories are negligible.

Leafy Vegetables		*Other vegetables*	
Bitter gourd (karela)	Curry leaves	Brinjal	Onion stalks
Amarnath	Fenugreek	Cauliflower	Pumpkin
Bathua	leaves	Cucumber	Radish
Brussels sprouts	Lettuce	Drumstick	Tinda
Cabbage	Mint	French beans	Tomato, Green
Celery	Spinach	Ladies Finger	Tumip
Coriander leaves	Soya Leaves	Mango, green	

For Persons Who do Strenuous Job (Hard Work)

2000 calories

SAMPLE MENU

	North	South	East	West
Pre-breakfast	1tea without Sugar	1 coffee without sugar	1tea without sugar	1 coffee or tea without sugar
	4 Marie &	6 banana chips	4 Marie &	4 Marie &
	2 Monaco biscuits	2 Monaco biscuits	2 Monaco biscuits	2 Monaco biscuits
	1/2 apple	1/2 small apple	1small orange	1 apple
Breakfast	4 slice bread	4 Idlies with chutney	4 slices bread	4 slices bread
	1teaspoon butter	1 teaspoon oil for cooking	1 teaspoon butter	1 teaspoon butter
	1 glass skimmed milk	1 glass skimmed milk	1 glass skimmed milk	1 glass skimmed milk
	2 eggs	2 eggs	2 eggs	2 eggs
Lunch	4-1/2 Chapaties	3 katories rice	3 Katories rice	1-1/2 chapaties and 2 katories rice
	1 Katori vegetable	1/2 katori sambar	1 katorie vegetable	1 Katorie vegetable
	2 teaspoon oil for cooking	2 teaspoon oil for cooking	2 teaspoon oil for cooking	2 teaspoon oil for cooking
	2/3 glass curd	2/3 glass curd	2/3 glass curd	2/3 glass curd
	3/4 Katori Rajmah	3/4 kator Lentils	3/4 Katori Lentils	3/4 Katori Lentils
Evening snack	1 tea without sugar	1 coffee without sugar	1 tea without sugar	1 coffee or tea without sugar
	4 Maire and	4 Maire and	4 Maire and	4 Maire and
	2 Monaco biscuits	2 Monaco biscuits	2 Monaco biscuits	2 Monaco biscuits
	1/2 apple	1/2 apple	2 piece orange	1/2 apple

Dinner

3 Chapaties+	2 Katories rice+	3 katories rice	11/2chapaties
1 katori rice	1-1/2 chapaties		& 2 chapaties
1Katori	1Katori	1katori	1Katori
vegetable	vegetable	vegetable	vegetable
1-1/2 teaspoon	1-1/2 teaspoon	1-1/2 teaspoon	1-1/2 teaspoon
oil	oil	oil	oil
for cooking	for cooking	for cooking	for cooking
1/3 glass curd	1/3 glass curd	1/3 glass curd	1/3 glass curd
1 piece chicken	1 piece chicken	1 piece fish	1 piece chicken

Food Values and General Guidelines.

Desserts*

	Household Measures	Wt/Vol	Calories
Custard		150gm	360
Fruits salad		150gm	150
Fruits Salad with cream		150gm	300
Ice, Cream		150 gm	380
Carrot halwa	1 medium katori	100 gm	600
Badami Halwa		100gm	570

Sweets*

	Household Measures	Wt/Vol	Calories
Coconut burfi		25gm	110
Gulabl Jamun		25gm	200
Ladoo		30gm	160
Rasgula		150 gm	140
Jam	2 table spoon		80
Honey	3 table spoon		48

Beverages**

		Wt/Vol	Calories
Beer		150ml	65
Wine dry		30ml	30
Wine dessert		30ml	40
Whisky, brandy, gin, rum		30ml	65
Vodka		30 ml	65
Ginger-etc.		30 ml	9

* It is better to avoid alcohol. Too much alcohol may cause low blood sugar by potentiating the effect of insulin or drugs and blocking glucose production in the liver while adding to calories. It can cause increase in cholesterol and triglycerides.

* Artificial sweetners like Aspartame and saccharine tables are available. They are safe and may be used in moderate amounts.
* Vegetables mentioned under the List 8 vegetable exchange have negligible calories and may be uséd whenever desirable.
* Avoid or restrict foodstuffs high in saturated fat and cholesterol.
* Avoid sweet foods, jams, chocolates, cakes, sweet cream, which increase triglyceride levels.
* Bake, roast, boil or steam instead of frying food.
* Do no replace oil and fat with calories in terms of sweets which when taken in excess gets converted to triglycerides.

Calorie Count/Content in Food

The nutritional unit of energy is calorie for the body. If food stuffs are not replaced in equal amount the body becomes thinner the quantity of calories per item are given below.

These are average figures, because the food values of raw materials can vary considerably.

Beverages

Beverages	Approximate Measures/Weight	Caloric Content (K Cal)
Aerated soft drinks	1 bottle	78
Lemonade	1 glass (250 ml.)	90
Fruit juices		
Apple	3/4 glass	87
Sweet Lime (fresh)	1glass	52
Orange (fresh)	1 glass	111
Pineapple (canned)	3/4 glass	104

Beverages	Approximate Measures/Weight	Caloric Content (K Cal)
Tomato (canned)	3/4 glass	34
Coconut water	1 coconut	120
Tea (clear, unsweetened)	1 cup (125ml.)	2
Coffee (clear, unsweetened)	1 cup	5
Chocolate (all milk)	1 glass	208
Bournvita powder	3 teaspoon full	88
Horlicks	5 teaspoon full	88
Protinex	2 teaspoon full	88
Soups		
Clear vegetable soup	1 cup	negligible
Chicken noodles soup	1 cup	59
Chicken soup	1 cup	75
Cream of tomato	1 cup	173
Cream of mushroom	1 cup	149
Cream of peas	1 cup	128
Alcoholic Beverages		
Beer	1 glass	114
Rum	1 jigger (45ml.)	105
Gin	I jigger (45ml.)	105
Whisky	1 jigger (45ml.)	105
Champagne	1 glass	84
Sherry	1 glass	84
Vodka	1 jigger (45ml.)	125

Cooked Food

Food	Approx. weight	Approx. Calories (K Cal)
Kacharui	100 gms.	500
Plain Dosa	100 gms.	360
Iddli	100 gms.	132
Pongal	100 gms.	356

Food	Approx. weight	Approx. Calories (K Cal)
Uthappam	100 gms.	330
Puri	40 gms.	184
Khichadi	100 gms.	168
Papdi Chat	100 gms.	474
Dhokla	100 gms.	122
Uppama	100 gms.	233
Poha	100 gms.	118
Muruku	100 gms.	529
Namkeen	100 gms.	521
Mathi	100 gms.	521
Samosa	100 gms.	256
Khakra	40 gms.	140
Adai	100 gms.	571
Aapam	100 gms.	226
Chiwda	100 gms.	420
Potato chips	20 gms.	113
Cheese Pizza	60 gms.	145
Ham Burger	90 gms.	244
Cheese Burger	100 gms.	290

Food	Calories/100gms. (K.cal.)
Bread	
Wholemeal	224
Granary white and brown	245-225.5
Cheese	
Cottage (low-fat)	105-115.5
Cream	445
Chutney	70-140

	Calories/100gms. *(K.cal.)*
Fats and oils	
Butter, margarine	738.5
Oils	892.5
Outline low fat spread	367.5
Fresh Fruits	
Apples, grapes, cherries	49
Soft fruit	21
Grapefruit	21
Melon	21
Orange, peaches	35
Pears, pineapples, plums	42
Fruit canned	77-105 (average)
Honey	287-315
Ice-cream	175
Jams	280 (average)
Fresh Meat	
Chicken	108.5
Liver	133
Pork	189
Milk	
Whole liquid	63
Dried skimmed	325.5
Soya liquid	35
Nuts, Shelled	
Brazil	630
Cashew	623
Coconut	343
Hazel	378
Peanuts	581
Walnuts	528.5
Nut, butter, peanut	630
Fresh vegetable	
Lettuce, mushroom celery	7
Sweedes, turnips	14

	Calories/100gms. (K.cal.)
Carrots, onions	21
Cauliflower, spring greens	25
Parsnips	45.5
Peas	63
Potatoes	84
Speas sweet corn	98
Wheat germ	350
Fruit-flavoured	77(average)

Calorie Consumption

Calorie Consumption	Body weight kgs.			
Per hour on the job	58	65	75	85
Driving (active)	204	228	252	276
Keyboarding	126	138	150	162
Managerial (desk sedentary)	204	228	252	276
Managerial (active)	222	246	270	294
Telephone Conversation	198	222	246	270
Teaching	204	228	252	276
Writing (sitting)	102	120	132	150
Exercising Badminton singles	312	348	384	420
Doubles	270	306	342	378
Dancing				
Aerobic (medium)	396	444	492	540
Contemporary (rock)	228	258	252	318
Golf				
Driving	228	258	228	318
Putting	138	156	174	192
Hill climbing	534	600	666	732
Running				
9 km/hr.	594	660	732	804
11 km/hr.	624	696	768	840
12 km/hr.	672	816	960	1104

Calorie Consumption	Body weight kgs.			
Per hour on the job	58	65	75	85
Swimming				
Slow	270	306	242	588
Medium	480	534	594	642
Fast	618	696	342	378
Tennis				
Singles	378	420	462	510
Doubles	270	306	342	378
Walking				
3.2 km./hr.	168	192	216	240
4.8 km./hr.	270	306	342	378
6.4 km.hr.	312	354	396	438
8 km./hr.	204	228	252	276
Yoga	204	228	252	276
Others				
Cooking	165	192	216	240
Card playing	90	102	114	132
Eating	84	90	96	102
Showering and dressing	180	204	228	252
Sitting quietly	72	84	96	108
Sitting talking	90	102	114	132
Sleeping	60	66	72	78
Waiting in line	90	102	114	132
Watching TV	78	90	96	102

Fruits to be avoided

Banana, Mango, Cheeku, Grapes, Sharifa should be avoided as they contain plenty of calories and sugar.

2. Cooking Oils

All cooking oils have same fat and calorie content but some may contain more fatty acids while other less.

Oils (fats) containing more saturated fatty acids should be avoided like *Vanaspati, coconut oil* and *margarine* should be avoided. While Ghee and butter may be used cautiously.

Oils which can be safely used.

Sunflower oil	Groundnut oil
Sunflower oil	Sesame oil
Corn oil	Soyabean oil

Foods to be avoided

Sugar and Gud
Jam, Candies
Choc Bar
Sweet, Achar-Pickles
Sonth
Beer, Whisky—Sherbat
Pineapple juice—tinned
Cold drinks
Boost, Maltova, Horlicks, Bournvita

Fruits permitted

Citrus fruits like Orange, Malta, Mosamabi, Kinnu, Grape fruit, Apple, Watermelon and Papaya can be taken. One can have one or two of the above fruits or above 100-150 gm. In case of watermelon one can have 400 gm as it contains plenty of water.

Height and Weight Table
Height (cm), Weight (kg.)— for Indian Males

Height (cm)	Age in years						
	20 kg	25 kg	30 kg	35 kg	40 kg	45 kg	50 kg
148	42.7	44.2	46.2	47.6	48.8	50.0	50.9
150	43.6	44.9	46.9	48.5	49.7	50.8	51.5
153	45.5	47.0	49.0	50.4	51.7	52.3	53.5
155	46.3	48.1	49.9	51.5	52.7	53.5	54.2
158	48.9	50.0	52.0	53.5	54.5	55.7	56.6
160	49.7	51.1	53.1	54.7	55.6	56.7	57.4
163	51.1	52.7	54.9	56.3	57.6	58.5	59.4
165	53.1	54.7	56.9	58.5	59.6	60.6	62.0
168	54.0	56.3	58.1	60.1	61.5	62.4	53.7
170	56.5	57.9	60.3	62.2	63.7	64.7	65.8
173	58.1	60.1	62.2	64.0	65.8	67.0	68.3
175	60.1	62.2	64.2	66.0	68.1	68.7	71.0
178	61.9	64.0	66.3	68.5	70.6	71.9	72.4
180	64.0	66.2	68.5	71.0	73.3	74.4	75.1
183	66.0	68.5	71.0	73.3	75.6	77.1	77.8
148	38.6	41.0	42.6	44.0	45.1	46.3	47.1
150	40.3	41.6	43.5	44.8	46.0	47.0	47.7
153	41.9	43.5	45.3	46.6	47.9	48.4	49.5
155	42.8	44.3	46.2	47.7	48.8	49.5	50.1
158	44.9	46.3	48.1	49.5	50.5	51.6	52.1
160	46.0	47.3	49.1	50.6	51.5	52.4	53.0
163	47.3	48.8	50.8	52.1	52.2	54.1	54.9
165	49.1	50.6	52.6	54.1	55.3	56.0	57.3
148	42.7	44.2	46.2	47.6	48.8	50.0	50.9
148	38.6	41.0	42.6	44.0	45.1	46.3	47.1
150	40.3	41.3	43.5	44.8	46.0	47.0	47.7
153	41.9	43.5	45.3	46.6	47.9	48.4	49.5
155	42.8	44.3	46.2	47.7	48.8	49.5	50.1
158	44.9	46.3	48.1	49.5	50.5	51.6	52.1
160	46.0	47.3	49.1	50.6	51.5	52.4	53.0
163	47.3	48.8	50.8	52.1	52.2	54.1	54.9

Calories Values

Breakfast Food

Foodstuff	Calories	Fat Saturated (gm)	Total (gm)	Cholesterol (mg)
Bacon Fried 1 slice (25gms)	95	2.8	9.0	3.0
Bread, White 2 Slice (40 gms)	98	-	0.3	-
Bun 1 big (60 gms)	170	-	0.4	-
Cheese Toast 2 Slice (70 gms)	220	8.0	13.1	19.5
Corn Flakes 1 cup without milk & sugar	95	-	Traces	-
Dosa—Masala/Mysore With butter (200 gms)	400	9.0	25.0	42.0
Dosa, Plain (50 gms)	200	7.0	10.0	-
Egg, White 1 white (17gms)	15	-	-	-
Egg Whole (50 gms)	87	1.7	6.6	248.0
Egg, Yolk 1 yolk (33gms)	62	1.7	6.6	248.0
Egg, Boiled (50 gms)	87	1.7	6.6	248.0
Egg (fried/omelet/scrambled)				
(a) suing 1 tbsp. (15 gm) butter/ghee	200	16.1	18.7	290.0
(b) using 1 tbsp Oil	225	11.2	21.6	248.0
Finger Chips 1 serving	465	21.0	30.2	-

Foodstuff	Calories	Fat Saturated (gm)	Total (gm)	Cholesterol (mg)
Fruit Bread 1 slice (20gms)	60	0.1	1.0	-
Ham, Roasted 1 slice (50 gms)	245	10.4	25.0	25.0
Idli with sambar (60gms)	250	1.0	5.0	-
Luncheon Meat 1 slice (20gms)	65	1.7	5.0	3.0
Milk bread 1 slice (20gms)	55	0.1	5.0	0.2
Milk, skimmed 1 cup (200ml)	74	-	0.2	0.4
Milk, whole 1 cup (200ml)	150	4.9	8.1	22.0
Phoe (Potato)	240	3.5	8.0	-
Parotha, Plain (50gms)	250	7.0	12.5	28.0
Parotha, stuffed (70gms)	300	7.0	12.5	28.0
Sausages, Cooked (25gms)	85	1.6	7.0	25.0
Salami 1 slice (10gms)	45	3.1	7.0	-
Tomato Omelet (60gms)	250	7.0	12.0	-
Uthappam, Onion (75gms)	275	7.0	10.8	-
Uppama 1 plate (150gms)	235	3.5	8.0	-

SNACKS 'N' SAVOURIES

Foodstuff	Calories	Fat Saturated (gm)	Total (gm)	Cholesterol (mg)
Belpuri 1 plate (150gms)	185	3.5	5.5	-
Biscuits, salted (10gms)	53	0.3	3.2	-

Foodstuff	Calories	Fat Saturated (gm)	Total (gm)	Cholesterol (mg)
Biscuits, Sweet (10gms)	45	0.1	1.3	-
Cutlets, Mutton (200gms)	480	18.5	28.5	95.0
Cutlets, Vegetable (200gms)	450	17.5	25.0	-
Dahiwada (200 gms)	250	10.5	19.5	-
Dalwada (60 gms)	340	9.0	15.0	-
Farsan/Chewada 1 plate (100gms)	230	10.5	15.0	-
Kachoris (150gms)	400	14.0	20.0	-
Patties (200gms)	300	7.0	10.0	-
Paneer pakoda (50gms)	275	15.2	22.0	20.0
Pizza (Meat) 1 small (225gms)	400	14.5	20.0	75.0
Pizza (Vegetable, Cheese) 1 small (200gms)	325	11.7	15.0	32.5
Potato Wadas (150gms)	470	14.0	20.0	-
Puri Bhaji 1 plate (250gms)	685	27.0	42.0	-
Ragada patties 1 plate (250gms)	450	7.0	13.0	-
Samosa (150gms)	500	14.0	20.0	-
Sev Puri 1 plate (200gms)	225	10.5	15.0	-
Bhajias, Onion 1 plate (150gms)	395	17.5	27.6	-
Cauliflower Pakoras 1 plate (150gms)	410	17.5	27.9	-

Foodstuff	Calories	Fat Saturated (gm)	Total (gm)	Cholesterol (mg)
Almonds (100gms)	655	4.2	58.9	-
Cashewnuts (100gms)	596	9.3	46.9	-
Pistachios (100gms)	680	7.8	57.8	-
Walnuts (100gms)	687	6.6	64.5	-

MEALS
a. Soups

Foodstuff	Calories	Fat Saturated (gm)	Total (gm)	Cholesterol (mg)
Chicken Soup 1 cup	185	6.8	12.5	87.0
Chicken Vegetable Soup 1 cup	162	4.4	8.7	73.0
Corn Soup (Sweet) 1 cup	120	1.7	7.0	248.0
Dal Soup 1 cup	137	2.2	4.2	14.0
Green Peas Soup 1 cup	176	2.2	5.5	14.0
Spinach Soup 1 cup	50	2.2	4.4	14.0
Tomato Soup 1 cup	87	2.2	4.2	14.0

Each cup equivalent to 200ml
b. Salads

Foodstuff	Calories	Fat Saturated (gm)	Total (gm)	Cholesterol (mg)
Russian Salad 1 serving (100gm)	545	18.1	50.0	289
Sprouted Pulse Salad 1 serving (100gm)	225	3.5	5.7	-

c. Vegetable

Foodstuff	Calories	Fat Saturated (gm)	Total (gm)	Cholesterol (mg)
Brinjal Bhartah 1 serving (150gm)	150	7.0	10.5	-
Chana Masala 1 serving (200gm)	240	7.0	10.0	-

Foodstuff	Calories	Fat Saturated (gm)	Total (gm)	Cholesterol (mg)
Chana Dal 1 bow/1 cup (150gms)	270	7.0	17.8	-
Dum Aloo 1 serving (150gm)	254	10.8	15.7	1.6
Macaroni & Tomato (butter) 1 serving (150gms)	396	15.4	27.3	70
Mixed Vegetables— Carrots Peas, Cauliflower, Beans etc. 1 serving (150gm)	175	7.0	10.5	-
Palak Paneer 1 serving (150gm)	180	11.0	13.0	20.0
Potato & Peas 1 serving (150gm)	235	7.0	10.0	-
Paneer Tikka 1 serving (150gm)	285	16.4	25.0	42.3
Potato Vegetable 1 serving (150gm)	165	7.0	11.2	-
MEALS **Dalbhaji (Spinach & Bengal Gram Dal)** 1 serving (150gm)	125	3.5	7.0	-
Stuffed Bhindi 1 serving (150gm)	200	3.5	6.2	-
Stuffed Capsicum (Simla Mirch) 1 serving (150gm)	120	3.5	6.0	-
Stuffed Karela 1 serving (150gm)	275	17.5	28.5	-
Usal 1 serving (150gm)	160	3.5	5.5	-
Vegetables, Leafy 1 serving (100gm)	100	3.5	5.5	-
Vegetables, Baked 1 serving (150gm)	395	6.7	22.5	5.3

Foodstuff	Calories	Fat Saturated (gm)	Total (gm)	Cholesterol (mg)
d. Cereals				
Bhakri (Jowar, Bajra, Ragi)	300	-	1.5	
1 med. (90gms)				
Biryani Mutton	255	11.5	16.5	
1 med. Bowl (150gms)				
Chappati	100	-	0.5	
1 med. (30 gms)				
Chappati with ghee 1 tsp	150	2.3	5.5	
1 med. (30 gms)				
Fired Rice	20	5.2	7.5	
1 med. Bowl (150 gms)				
Khichadi	190	3.5	10.0	
1 serving (150 gms)				
Naan	225	2.1	3.4	
1 no. (20gms)				
Puris	105	4.2	6.2	
1 no. (20 gms)				
Pulao, Vegetable	170	3.5	5.0	
1 med. Bowl (100gms)				
Rice cooked	100	-	-	
1 med. Bowl (100gms)				
Khadi	150	7.5	11.0	2.7
1 bow/cup (200ml)				
Kofta Curry	225	10.0	15.0	
1 serving (200ml)				
Lauki Dal	150	7.0	11.5	
1 bowl/cup (200ml)				
Rajma Curry	290	7.0	10.7	
1 bowl/cup (200ml)				
Prawn Pulao	510	7.3	32.5	150
1 serving				
Egg Fried Rice	280	1.7	16.7	248
1 serving				

Foodstuff	Calories	Fat Saturated (gm)	Total (gm)	Cholesterol (mg)
NON-VEGETARIAN				
Beef Curry	185	8.0	11.0	100
1 serving				
Chicken Butter	305	11.4	21.0	160
1 serving				
Chicken Curry	175	7.1	10.4	70
1 serving				
Chicken Chilli	255	10.5	16.0	90
1 serving				
Chicken Fried in	440	15.0	25.5	217
Butter 1 serving				
Chicken Paella	325	10.5	15.8	45
1 serving				
Chicken Patties	335	14.0	20.4	45
2 pieces				
Chopsuey	150	7.3	11.4	18
1 serving				
Egg Curry	235	12.4	21.5	248
1 serving				
Elaichi Mutton	215	1.5	13.6	70
1 serving				
Fish Baked	395	8.7	32.3	107
1 serving				
Fish Curry	35	3.5	7.0	50
1 serving				
Fish & Chips	850	35.2	52.8	130
1 serving				
Fish in Curds (Hilsa)	505	14.5.	40.5	82
1 serving				
Fish Fried	220	10.5	17.5	50
1 piece (50 gms)				
Kheema Mutton	240	8.5	13.6	70
1 serving				
Mutton Curry	185	8.0	12.7	95
1 serving				

Foodstuff	Calories	Fat Saturated (gm)	Total (gm)	Cholesterol (mg)
Mutton Vindaloo 1 serving	334	18.5	28.6	70
Nargisi Kabab 2 pieces	360	17.0	29.3	301
Pork Curry 1 serving	185	8.3	13.5	80
Pork Sorpote (Goan) 1 serving	321	15.4	25.1	165
Prawns Fried 1 serving	273	14.1	21.0	150
Prawn Malaya Curry 1 serving	415	28.0	32.4	150
Stewed Mutton 1 serving	145	4.5	7.5	95
Stuffed Mutton Malai Kofta 1 serving	600	27.0	50.0	215
Sweet & Sour Mutton 1 serving	285	10.5	20.5	176

Note: Each serving equivalent to 150 gms unless indicated otherwise.

ORGAN MEAT				
Brain (100gms)	107	2.4	8.5	2235
Heart Beef, Goat (100gms)	115	1.5	5.0	256
Kidney Goat (100gms)	120	4.2	11.0	700
Liver				
Beef (100gms)	110	2.6	5.3	406
Goat (100gms)	107	2.6	5.3	406
Lamb (100gms)	110	2.8	6.8	510
Pork (100gms)	110	2.9	5.5	420
SEA FOOD				
Crabs Cooked (75gms raw)	155	-	10.5	70

Foodstuff	Calories	Fat Saturated (gm)	Total (gm)	Cholesterol (mg)
Prawns, Cooked (75gms raw)	155	-	10.5	70
Lobsters (75gms raw)	165	-	12.0	70
SWEETS & DESSERTS				
Amriti (50gms)	295	10.5	16.0	-
Basundi 1 serving (150gms)	270	6.0	12.0	27.5
Besan Ladoo (50gms)	205	5.5	8.5	-
Bundi Ladoo (50gms)	210	5.2	8.5	-
Cake, Iced 1 slice (55 gms)	190	4.8	8.0	50.0
Cake, Plain 1 slice (40 gms)	118	1.0	2.5	30.0
Cake, Fruit 1 slice (40 gms)	155	3.6	6.2	30.0
Custard, Plain 1 serving (200gms)	220	5.0	8.2	22.0
Custard with Jelly 1 serving (225gms)	230	5.0	8.2	22.0
Fruit Salad 1 serving (225gms)	250	5.0	8.2	22.0
Gulab Jamun (60gms)	282	13.0	20.2	12.5
Halwa, Vegetable (carrot, pumpkin, gourd) 1 serving (200gms)	225	7.0	13.7	42.0
Ice-Cream (Small) 1 cup (100gms)	215	6.7	10.8	45.0
Jalebi (40gms)	280	10.5	16.0	-

Foodstuff	Calories	Fat Saturated (gm)	Total (gm)	Cholesterol (mg)
Kheer, Rice 1 avg. serving (200gms)	240	3.6	8.0	22.0
Kheer, Vermicelli 1 serving (200gms)	240	3.6	8.5	22.0
Modak, Fried (50 gms)	250	11.0	19.5	-
Modak Steamed (40gms)	160	5.2	9.4	-
Pudding, Bread 1 serving (150gms)	300	7.0	15.3	5.0
Pudding, Milk 1 serving (150gms)	280	7.0	14.8	58.0
Puran Poli (60gms)	315	14.0	26.0	-
Rasgulla (40gms)	180	2.4	4.2	7.0
Rewal Ladoo (50gms)	205	5.2	8.5	-
Rasmalai, 2 Rasgullas 1 serving (150gms)	370	9.6	12.5	29.0

Foodstuff	Calories	Fat	Prot.	Carbohyd.
		(gm)	(gm)	(gm)
Almonds (100gms)	655			
Cashewnuts (100gms)	596		109	
Pistachios (100gm)			178	
Walnots (100gm)	687	545		
MEATS				
a. Soups				
Chicken Soup 1 cup	185	8.6	12.6	33.0
Chicken Vegetable Soup 1 cup	162	4.3		
Corn Soup (Sweet) 1 cup	220		10.9	36.00
Dal Soup 1 cup	72			14.0
Green Peas Soup 1 cup	156	2.2		18.0
Spinach Soup 1 cup	76	2.2		14.0
Potato Soup 1 cup	157		4.0	16.0
Each cup equivalent to 100ml				
b. Salads				
Russian Salad 1 serving (100gm)	346	14.4	30.0	7.0
Sprouted Pulse Salad 1 serving (100gm)	225	2.2	4.7	
c. Vegetable				
Brinjal Bhartha 1 serving (130gm)	150	2.0	10.5	
Chana Masala 1 serving (100gm)	240	2.0	10.0	